Venous Thromboembolism in Advanced Disease
A Clinical Guide

Edited by

Simon I.R. Noble
Clinical Senior Lecturer and
Honorary Consultant in Palliative Medicine
Cardiff University and the Royal Gwent Hospital
Newport, Wales, UK

Miriam J. Johnson
Senior Lecturer in Palliative Medicine
Hull York Medical School and Honorary Consultant to
St Catherine's Hospice and Scarborough and North East Yorkshire
Health Care Trust, UK

Agnes Y.Y. Lee
Medical Director of Thrombosis
Division of Hematology
Vancouver Coastal Health and Vancouver Acute
Vancouver, BC;
Associate Professor
Department of Medicine
University of British Columbia
Vancouver, BC;
Clinical Associate Professor
Department of Medicine
McMaster University
Hamilton, ON, Canada

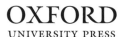

OXFORD
UNIVERSITY PRESS

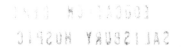

OXFORD
UNIVERSITY PRESS

Great Clarendon Street, Oxford OX2 6DP

Oxford University Press is a department of the University of Oxford.
It furthers the University's objective of excellence in research, scholarship,
and education by publishing worldwide in

Oxford New York

Auckland Cape Town Dar es Salaam Hong Kong Karachi
Kuala Lumpur Madrid Melbourne Mexico City Nairobi
New Delhi Shanghai Taipei Toronto

With offices in

Argentina Austria Brazil Chile Czech Republic France Greece
Guatemala Hungary Italy Japan Poland Portugal Singapore
South Korea Switzerland Thailand Turkey Ukraine Vietnam

Oxford is a registered trade mark of Oxford University Press
in the UK and in certain other countries

Published in the United States
by Oxford University Press Inc., New York

British Library Cataloguing in Publication Data
Data available

Library of Congress Cataloging-in-Publication-Data
Data available

Typeset by Cepha Imaging Private Ltd., Bangalore, India
Printed in the UK
on acid-free paper by
the MPG Books Group

ISBN 978-0-19-923204-8

10 9 8 7 6 5 4 3 2 1

Foreword

Thromboembolism has been greatly under-recognized in clinical practice. The editors have become leaders in the field of thrombosis and embolism in advanced disease and research in the complexities of thrombotic events is now impacting on clinical care and decision-making. Under diagnosis and misdiagnosis of emboli, particularly pulmonary embolic phenomena has meant that dyspnoea in many patients was probably in part avoidable. But today, despite anticoagulation, there are still fatalities.

The mechanisms behind the anticoagulant resistance, sensitivity, and the labile response seen to warfarin in cancer patients have eluded most clinicians in oncology and palliative care.

There is no other text like this available. This book, written in accessible yet scientific terms, will potentially educate clinicians and result in improved clinical decision-making. It should also inspire further research.

The beneficiaries are the patients and their families who entrust us, as clinicians, with their lives. Those lives should not be foreshortened by avoidable thromboembolism. This book is key in changing the pattern of disease.

Professor the Baroness Ilora Finlay of Llandaff

Preface

Venous thromboembolism (VTE) is a significant and common problem in patients with cancer and other medical conditions. It can be difficult to manage in patients with advanced disease. Whilst the recommendations for the management of VTE within the general medical population are based on strong research evidence, such research has involved few patients with life-limiting disease.

Unique challenges face the clinician looking after patients with advanced disease and VTE. The clinician must apply the best available evidence in the context of the individual, whilst weighing up the impact such treatment may have on the patients' quality of life.

This book brings together some of the leading figures from the worlds of VTE and palliative care to provide practical, evidence-based strategies to address some of the current knowledge gaps that exist in this specialized, yet clinically common area. Taking the current evidence, the authors have applied it to the management of patients with advanced disease in several settings, including the hospice, home, or acute care hospital. Specific chapters highlighting the management of advanced non-malignant disease and clinical decision-making in advanced disease are also included.

As well as being a practical aid to the care of patients, it is hoped that this book will stimulate and inspire further research into the management of VTE in advanced disease. Recognizing and addressing the unmet clinical needs of this special population is long overdue. We hope you will enjoy this book as much as we have enjoyed putting it together.

Simon I.R. Noble
Miriam J. Johnson
Agness Y.Y. Lee

Contents

Contributors

Aneel A. Ashrani
Assistant Professor of Medicine,
Division of Hematology,
Department of Internal Medicine,
Mayo Clinic College of Medicine,
Rochester, MN, USA

Sara Booth
Macmillan Consultant in Palliative
Care, Addenbrooke's Palliative Care
Team, Cambridge, UK

Dawn Dowding
Senior Lecturer in Clinical
Decision Making, Department of
Health Sciences, University of York
and Hull York Medical School, UK

Sarah J. Lewis
Consultant Haematologist and Lead
Clinician for Thrombosis, Royal
Gwent Hospital, Newport, UK

John A. Heit
Director, Thrombophilia Center,
General and Special Coagulation
Laboratories, and the Special
Coagulation DNA Diagnostic
Laboratory, Mayo Clinic;
Professor of Medicine, Divisions
of Cardiovascular Diseases and
Hematology, Department of
Internal Medicine, Mayo Clinic
College of Medicine,
Rochester, MN, USA

Menno V. Huisman
Department of General Internal
Medicine, Leiden University
Medical Center, The Netherlands

Beverley J. Hunt
Department of Haematology,
St Thomas's Hospital,
London, UK

Miriam J. Johnson
Senior Lecturer in Palliative
Medicine, Hull York Medical School
and Honorary Consultant to
St Catherine's Hospice, Scarborough,
and North East Yorkshire Health
Care Trust, UK

Agnes Y.Y. Lee
Medical Director of Thrombosis,
Division of Hematology, Vancouver
Coastal Health and Vancouver Acute;
Associate Professor, Department of
Medicine, University of British
Columbia, Vancouver, BC;
Associate Clinical Professor,
Department of Medicine, McMaster
University, Hamilton, ON, Canada

Simon I.R. Noble
Clinical Senior Lecturer and
Honorary Consultant in Palliative
Medicine, Cardiff University and the
Royal Gwent Hospital, Newport, UK

Anna Spathis
Locum Consultant in Palliative
Medicine, Oxfordshire, UK

Robert Weinkove
Department of Haematology,
St Thomas's Hospital, London, UK

Chapter 1

The challenge for palliative care

Simon I.R. Noble and Miriam J. Johnson

The changing role of palliative care

For the past 40 years, we have seen many fundamental changes in the management of patients with advanced disease. The modern hospice movement—from which the speciality of palliative care evolved—originally focussed on the end-of-life care of people with incurable cancer. Funded by the voluntary sector, hospices existed as standalone facilities often some distance—both geographically and philosophically—from mainstream and acute medicine. The complex symptoms of incurable disease do not manifest themselves solely at the end of life; they may be present throughout the disease including times of active dissease management. It has been recognized that palliative care services must adopt a model that integrates the philosophy of holistic symptom management alongside mainstream medicine. For many healthcare professionals, doctors in particular, the death of a patient is considered a failure and can sometimes inhibit the transition of active therapy to care directed primarily at symptom control. However, just as practitioners in mainstream medicine need to become more open to this culture shift and become proficient in the generic palliative care skills required to manage progressive life-limiting illness when it becomes unresponsive to curative measures, there is also a need for palliative care professionals to maintain a level of acute medical knowledge and skills in a rapidly changing environment in order to identify when patients have reversible pathology to account for their deterioration.

There are several factors that have driven the expansion of palliative care beyond just the provision of terminal care for cancer patients. The advances in the management of metastatic diseases including breast, colorectal, and urological cancers imply patients can live long with incurable cancer and may receive palliative anticancer therapies for several years. The natural history of cancer is changing and the metastatic disease has become, for many patients, a chronic illness, with palliative therapies continuing several years beyond the diagnosis of the incurable disease. Forty years ago, therapeutic options were limited for these patients making prognostication and care planning more predictable. As long as we have more therapies available to them, patients have better access to information and different expectations.

Although the association between venous thromboembolism (VTE) and cancer has been recognized for over 140 years, it is only in the last 15 years that it has been explored in the palliative care literature. To date fewer than twenty original papers have been published specific to palliative care populations. Whilst there appear to be particular challenges to the management of VTE in the palliative care setting, one must remember that palliative care teams manage only a small proportion of patients with advanced disease; the majority are cared for by oncologists, general physicians, and family doctors.

Definition of patient population

Whilst this book purports to consider VTE in advanced diseases, it raises challenges in defining what one means by a 'palliative care patient' or someone with 'advanced disease'. There is no agreed definition of a palliative care patient although various suggestions have been made.[1] Defining a patient as palliative based on predicted prognosis is one possibility, for example an estimated prognosis of less than 6 months. However, doctors have shown to be overoptimistic in their estimation of survival and as discussed before, people are living longer with metastatic disease requiring symptom-control measures for longer.

For cancer patients, the presence of metastatic disease could be an appropriate reference point from which to define the disease as palliative or advanced. In practice, with increasing therapies available for patients with metastases, patients are likely to remain under the main care of oncology teams for years. Considering the World Health Organization's definition of palliative care, the speciality looks after 'patients facing problems associated with life-threatening illness'.[2] By this definition, not every patient with terminal disease needs palliative care and the service will focus on those with the most complex needs.

For the purpose of this book, a palliative care patient will be defined as someone with disease which is no longer amenable to cure. The majority of chapters will focus on incurable cancer patients, which may be a heterogeneous group of varied performance statuses, prognoses, and degrees of metastatic disease. It includes those who despite having liver or brain metastases may still have good performance status as well as those who are asymptomatic but of performance status 3 or 4. However, as Chapter 2 highlights, healthcare professionals are looking after an increasing number of elderly patients in hospitals, nursing homes, hospices, and via home care services. As a patient's age increases, so too does the burden of complex and multiple comorbidities and pathologies. For this reason, VTE in the non-cancer population shall be explored in Chapter 9.

Underrecognition of VTE in advanced disease

Despite a suggested prevalence of asymptomatic VTE in over 50 per cent of palliative care patients, the perceived incidence is considerably smaller at around 1–5 per cent.[3–6] Palliative care physicians, whilst recognizing the thrombogenicity of malignant disease, do not consider it a major problem in the palliative care inpatient setting.[7] There may be several reasons for this. First, the true natural history of asymptomatic VTE in the palliative care patient is not known. It is possible that not all thrombi will progress to symptoms and, therefore, cause no problems. Second, the reported incidence may represent an underappreciation of the risk factors of advanced malignancy amongst palliative care physicians. The practice of VTE management varies worldwide and risks of VTE with cancer are underappreciated by least 25 per cent of oncologists.[8,9]

The common presenting symptoms of VTE are similar to those of other common pathologies experienced by patients with advanced cancer. For example, a painful swollen leg raises a high index of suspicion in a non-cancer patient whilst there are several causes to consider in the palliative care setting. Likewise dyspnoea, the commonest symptom associated with pulmonary embolism (PE), is seen in many common conditions associated with advanced cancer. It is important to recognize that although many conditions may mimic VTE, the presence of one such diagnosis does not negate the concurrent diagnosis of thrombosis. Acute conditions such as infection, heart failure, and local venous obstruction will increase the prothrombotic state and likelihood of undiagnosed VTE.[10]

Finally, there remains a perception that, even if someone has a high clinical suspicion of having VTE, it will be challenging to treat safely and alter the ultimate outcome of a 'terminally ill' patient. If one is unsure about the appropriateness of treating a problem, they will be less inclined to investigate it. These issues shall be covered in Chapter 8.

Confirmation of VTE

As a patient's treatment moves from active care to an approach focussed more on symptom control, the quality of life impact of investigations and the management of conditions the tests may uncover become more important and will contribute to decision-making. Simple exclusory tests such as the use of

D-dimers have a limited role in patients with malignant disease (discussed further in Chapter 4) and ventilation perfusion scans are of little help in those with known lung pathology.[11] For specialist palliative care unit inpatients, which are commonly located in separate units—often geographically some distance from radiology departments—accessing appropriate radiology such as computer tomograms and Doppler ultrasound, many cause logistical challenges and in some patients it may be considered inappropriate to transfer them for investigation. The same problem may be an issue for a patient wishing to remain at home.

The choice of investigation may require careful consideration as well. Investigations such as ventilation perfusion scan, which have an established role in the diagnosis of suspected PE in the general population, will be less appropriate in patients with additional lung pathology. Other investigations, which require the patient to lie flat for a period of time, may not be possible due to pain or dyspnoea.

Anticoagulation

In addition to being at high risk of developing VTE, advanced cancer patients are at greater risk of bleeding complications whilst anticoagulated[12–14] (discussed more fully in Chapter 6). The advanced cancer population is highly heterogeneous with respect to bleeding risk. Primary tumours including gastric, bladder, and lung cancer often present with bleeding problems and are a particular challenge when weighing up risks and benefits of treating VTE. Likewise, patients with highly vascular cerebral metastatic disease (e.g., thyroid, renal, melanoma) are at risk of intracranial haemorrhage on anticoagulation. Furthermore, patients with cancer and VTE are at high risk of developing recurrent VTE despite anticoagulation. Since the prothrombotic state increases with disease progression, it is likely that the risk of recurrent VTE increases as well. Treatment of such patients is especially difficult since increasing the dose of anticoagulant in order to control the resistant thrombotic process will necessarily increase the bleeding risk as well.

Alternative interventions to or concurrent with anticoagulation such as vena caval filters may be an option for some although the risks, benefits, and costs must be considered carefully when using them in a patient group of limited life expectancy and there is little evidence to guide the clinician in their use.

Paternalistic nihilism

The management of VTE in advanced disease is controversial, especially the issue of primary thromboprophylaxis in the inpatient setting. Some of this is driven by a genuine belief that there is insufficient evidence to justify certain therapies, and for others VTE prevention may appear countercultural to the palliative care philosophy. More concerning is a perception that VTE is 'a nice way to go' implying that a sudden painless death would be a preferable death to other terminal events. This opinion relies on the belief that fatal pulmonary emboli are both symptom-free and occur without warning. The published literature would suggest these beliefs are untrue. In a study of 92 patients, where PE was confirmed at autopsy as the cause of death, only 27 patients (30 per cent) died within 10 minutes of the onset of symptoms. Of these, only nine died abruptly with no preceding symptoms.[15] The clinical experience of patients taking longer than ten minutes to die was of a 'gradual deterioration dominated by dyspnoea, tachycardia, and fever'. A correct diagnosis of PE was made in only ten per cent of patients with most being treated with diuretics, digoxin, and antibiotics for presumed infection or heart failure. The evidence from this study suggests that in the majority of patients who died from a PE, the death was neither sudden nor symptom-free. In addition, the diagnosis was not made in 90 per cent of cases and so appropriate treatment and symptom control was not given. Furthermore, even if sudden death from VTE were sudden and painless, the patient may not wish this if given an informed choice. In circumstances where patients are at risk of preventable VTE, it would seem in keeping with palliative care philosophy to involve patients in such a decision.

Poor evidence base

The evidence base for treatment and prevention of VTE in metastatic disease is lacking and the best practice is guided by the extrapolation of data from studies in other populations. Even when reviewing robust studies in similar populations, the recorded outcome measures may be less relevant to palliative patients. For example, most studies will divide bleeding complications into major (causing death, requiring transfusion, bleeding into vital organ) or minor (everything else). These definitions, whilst useful as safety data, do not take into account the patient perspective or quality of life. A bleeding complication may be classified as minor by research criteria, but may be highly distressing for a vulnerable patient. There are several anticoagulants to choose from, although they differ in their efficacy, safety, drug interaction, cost, evidence base in cancer, and ease of administration. For some, anticoagulation will be too burdensome when compared with potential benefits.

Absence of guidelines in advanced disease

The paucity of evidence specific to the advanced disease population makes the production of high-quality guidelines difficult. The absence of robust studies in the palliative setting, and the heterogeneous population make it difficult to offer a 'one size fits all' recommendation. However, guidelines for the primary and secondary prevention of VTE in the general and cancer population are available and offer some assistance in the management of patients with incurable disease.

Education

With the recognition of palliative care as a specialty, acknowledgement has come that certain aspects of advanced disease management require specialist knowledge and skills. As with all specialties, the knowledge base of palliative care is continually increasing as more research is undertaken. However, most palliative care is provided by general healthcare professionals and family practitioner teams. Such specialist knowledge needs to be disseminated rather than remain in the specialist literature. Educational needs should be addressed not only at undergraduate level but continued throughout the postgraduate career as life-long professional development.

Research

The challenges of conducting research in the palliative care setting has been recognized for some time now and the poor evidence base for VTE management in the palliative care setting reflects this.[16] Conducting a robust clinical study into the treatment or prevention of VTE in palliative care patients would be a considerable undertaking and would require large-scale collaboration. In addition, it would need experienced clinical trials infrastructure to coordinate the study with additional research staff support at clinical sites and sufficient funding to do this. Until this occurs, best practice should be based on emerging trials within the surgical and medical populations.

Conclusions

Advances in healthcare have helped the population live longer, yet with longevity has come an increase in the burden of chronic disease. The model of palliative care has changed over time, and with this change, there has been an increase in the range of conditions and problems considered appropriate for palliative care intervention. The appreciation of the burden of VTE in advanced disease is developing, as is the evidence base by which clinicians are guided. It is becoming more appropriate to treat VTE in advanced disease and the prevention of VTE, whilst controversial, may have a place in specific patient groups. The major challenge now is how to apply the current evidence to patients with advanced disease, to ensure they receive appropriate VTE management that maximizes their quality of life and is in accordance with their wishes.

References

1. Maltoni M, Caraceni A, Brunelli C *et al.* Prognostic factors in advanced cancer patients: evidence based clinical recommendations–a study by the Steering Committee of the European Association for Palliative Care. *Journal of Clinical Oncology* 2005;23(25):6240–8.

2. World Health Organization. Definition of palliative care. www.who.int/cancer/palliative/definition/en/ (accessed 2008 Feb 12).

3. Johnson MJ, Sproule MW, Paul J. The prevalence and associated variables of deep venous thrombosis in patients with advanced cancer. *Clinical Oncology* 1999;11:105–10.

4. Ambrus JL, Ambrus CM, Pickren JW. Causes of death in cancer patients. *Journal of Medicine* 1975;6:61–4.

5. Sproul EE. Carcinoma and venous thrombosis: the frequency of association of carcinoma in the body or tail of the pancreas with multiple venous thrombosis. *American Journal of Cancer* 1938;34:566–85.

6. Johnson MJ, Sherry K. How do palliative physicians manage venous thromboembolism? *Palliative Medicine* 1997 Nov;11(6):462–8.

7. Noble SIR, Nelson A, Finlay IG. Factors influencing hospice thromboprophylaxis policy: a qualitative study. *Palliative Medicine* 2008;22:3 (abstract).

8. Wolf RA. Are patients with cancer receiving adequate thromboprophylaxis? Results from FRONTLINE. *Cancer Treatment Reviews* 2003 Jun;29(Suppl 2):7–9.

9. Kirwan CC. Prophylaxis for venous thromboembolism during treatment for cancer: questionnaire survey. *British Medical Journal* 2003;327:597, 598.

10. Noble SIR. Challenges in the management of venous thrombosis in the palliative care setting. *Postgraduate Medical Journal* 2007;83:671–4.

11. Hull RD, Hirsh J, Carter CJ *et al.* Diagnostic value of ventilation-perfusion lung scanning in patients with suspected pulmonary embolism. *Chest* 1985 Dec;88(6):819–28.

12. Hutten BA, Prins MH, Gent M *et al.* Incidence of recurrent thromboembolic and bleeding complications among patients with venous thromboembolism in relation to both malignancy and achieved international normalized ratio: a retrospective analysis. *Journal of Clinical Oncology* 2000;18:3078–83.

13. Prandoni P. Antithrombotic strategies in patients with cancer. *Thrombosis and Haemostasis* 1997;78(suppl):141–4.

14. Johnson MJ. Problems of anticoagulation within a palliative care setting: an audit of hospice patients taking warfarin. *Palliative Medicine* 1997 Jul;11(4):306–12.

15. Havig O. Deep vein thrombosis and pulmonary embolism: an autopsy study with multiple regression analysis of possible risk factors. *Acta Chirurgica Scandinavica Supplementum* 1977;478:1–120.

16. Keeley PW, Waterhouse ET, Noble SIR. The evidence base of palliative medicine: is inpatient palliative medicine evidence based? *Palliative Medicine* 2007;21(7):623–7.

Chapter 2

Epidemiology of venous thromboembolism

Aneel A. Ashrani and John A. Heit

Introduction

Venous thromboembolism (VTE), comprising deep vein thrombosis (DVT) and pulmonary embolism (PE), is a relatively common and frequently lethal disease. It is a multifactorial disease, involving interactions between environmental exposures and genetic predispositions. About one-third of the surviving cases have a recurrent VTE episode and an equal proportion develop its long-term sequel, venous stasis syndrome. Both the risk of VTE and the risk of death following VTE are dramatically increased in elderly individuals. Owing to longer life spans and the aging 'baby boom' generation, the average age of the population is increasing. By 2030, those over 75 years of age will account for 20 per cent of the population.[1] Moreover, elderly individuals are at markedly increased risk of hospitalization and nursing home (NH) admission, both known risk factors for VTE.[2,3] Data from the United States identifies the leading causes for hospitalization in the elderly population are congestive heart failure, pneumonia, joint replacement surgery, and chronic obstructive lung disease (COPD) exacerbation, all of which are associated risk factors of VTE.[4] There is also an increasing utilization of skilled nursing facilities, home health agencies, and hospice care.[4] Most NH residents suffer from multiple conditions. According to most recent figures from the National Long-Term Care Survey (NLTCS), 46 per cent of NH residents in 1999 who were admitted in a hospital were treated under acute and/or chronic medical conditions.[5] These high levels of morbidity were accompanied by substantial disability; 75 per cent of NH residents were dependent for three or more activities of daily living (ADLs), that is, bathing, eating, dressing, etc., and 69 per cent were dependent for five to six ADLs.[5] Utilization of skilled nursing and home health services has been increasing (Fig. 2.1), indicating an increase in the burden of chronic medical diseases in the population. Despite the increase in the utilization of prophylactic measures for prevention of VTE (albeit still underutilized), the

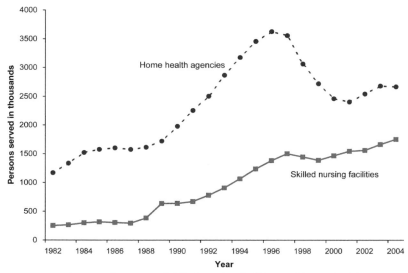

Fig. 2.1 Trends in Medicare use of skilled nursing facilities and home health agencies.[4]

incidence of VTE over the years has remained relatively unchanged.[6] As the average age of the population increases, the total number of VTE events (and associated deaths) occurring each year will likely increase. Therefore, prevention of VTE in individuals at increased risk (i.e., the elderly population and individuals with advanced diseases) could contribute to a marked reduction in the overall burden of VTE. Better individual risk stratification is needed in order to target primary and secondary VTE prophylaxis to individuals who would benefit the most. This review focuses on the disease burden (incidence), outcomes (survival, recurrence, and complications) and risk factors of VTE in the community, the elderly population, and in individuals with advanced diseases.

VTE: the disease burden

The overall average age- and sex-adjusted incidence of VTE is about 1.2–1.9 per 1000 person-years.[6] The incidence of VTE has remained unchanged over the last few decades (Fig. 2.2) despite introduction of more effective prophylaxis regimens for prevention of VTE and an increase in the utilization of these prophylactic measures.[6] Compared to the 10-year period, 1981–1990, when the incidence of VTE was 116 per 100,000 person-years, the incidence for the subsequent 9-year period, 1991–1999, remained virtually unchanged at 118 per 100,000 person-years. This relative constant VTE incidence could reflect an increase in the population at risk (e.g., increase in the average age of

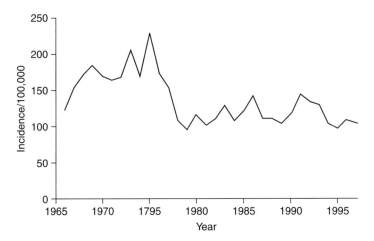

Fig. 2.2 Trends in VTE incidence: 1966–1997.[6] Reproduced with permission from *Archives of Internal Medicine* 1998;158:585–93. Copyright American Medical Association. All rights reserved.

the population,[1] or exposure to more or new risk factors (e.g., increase in the surgical procedures;[7] increase in NH admissions[4]). As the average age of the population increases, the total number of VTE events (and associated deaths) occurring each year will increase likely.

The incidence varies markedly depending on an individual's age and sex (Figs. 2.3 and 2.4). For example, the incidence of VTE among individuals 14 years old or younger is less than 1 per 100,000 person-years. The incidence begins to increase dramatically in the fifth decade of life; therefore for 80-year-olds or older, the incidence approaches 1 per 100 person-years.[6] The higher risk of VTE associated with advancing age may be due to the

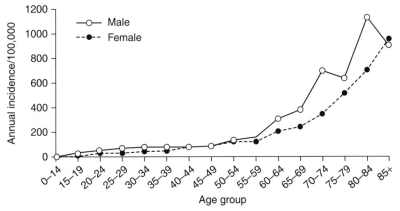

Fig. 2.3 Annual incidence of VTE by age and gender.[6] Reproduced with permission from *Archives of Internal Medicine* 1998;158:585–93. Copyright American Medical Association. All rights reserved.

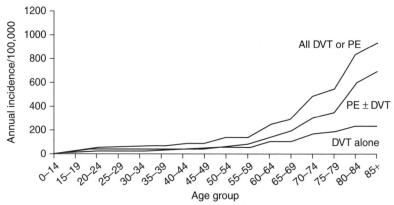

Fig. 2.4 Annual incidence of all VTE, DVT alone, and PE with or without DVT (PE ± DVT) by age and VTE type.[6] Reproduced with permission from *Archives of Internal Medicine* 1998;158:585–93. Copyright American Medical Association. All rights reserved.

biology of aging rather than simply an increased exposure to VTE risk factors with advancing age.[8] The incidence is higher among women during child-bearing years because of the risk factors associated with reproduction (i.e., oral contraceptives, pregnancy, and puerperium), while the incidence is higher among men above 50 years of age.[6] PE accounts for an increasing proportion of VTE with increasing age for both genders.[6] Hence, as the average population age increases, the total number of incident VTE events per year will increase, and an increasing number of these events will be PE.

The incidence of VTE also varies by race. Compared to whites, African-Americans have a slightly higher VTE incidence (hazard ratio [HR] 1.27), while Asian- and Native-Americans have a dramatically lower VTE incidence (HR 0.26), the incidence among Hispanics is intermediate between whites and Asian-Americans (HR 0.6).[9,10] Based on the above rates, it has been estimated that over 275,000 incident VTE cases occur annually in the US residents. Using an incidence-based model that included both hospital- and community-acquired VTE events as well as death from recognized and unrecognized VTE, it is conservatively estimated that over 900,000 US residents develop incident or recurrent VTE each year; almost one-third of these cases are fatal.[11]

VTE outcomes

Mortality

The survival following VTE is much worse than the age- and sex-matched expected survival, and the survival after PE is much worse than after DVT alone.[12,13] Overall, about 30 per cent of VTE patients die within

Table 2.1 Survival after first lifetime DVT alone, PE with our without DVT (PE ± DVT), and all VTE.[12] Reproduced with permission from *Archives of Internal Medicine* 1999;1598:445–58. Copyright American Medical Association. All rights reserved.

Time	DVT alone (per cent)	PE ± DVT		All VTE (per cent)
		All PE (per cent)	PE as cause of death (per cent)	
0 days	97.0	63.6	76.5	77.7
7 days	96.2	59.1	71.1	74.8
14 days	95.7	57.1	68.7	73.3
30 days	94.5	55.6	66.8	72.0
90 days	91.1	52.1	62.8	68.9
1 year	85.4	47.7	57.4	63.6
2 years	81.4	44.6	53.6	60.1
5 years	72.6	39.4	47.4	53.5
8 years	65.2	34.5	41.5	47.5

3 months of diagnosis (Table 2.1).[12] The risk of early death among PE patients is as high as 18 when compared to DVT patients alone. Almost one-quarter of PE cases die suddenly without forewarning or seeking medical attention, and almost 40 per cent die within 3 months. VTE often affects individuals with other concurrent diseases that reduce survival. However, after controlling other common medical causes of death, PE independently reduces survival for up to 3 months.[12]

Independent predictors of decreased 7-day survival after VTE include increasing age, male gender, lower body mass index (BMI), confinement to a hospital or nursing home at the onset of VTE, and a history of congestive heart failure (CHF), chronic lung disease, serious neurological disease, and malignancy (Table 2.2).[12] Thus, ill-health, as evident by a BMI below normal or confinement to a hospital or nursing home, predicted lower survival after controlling other debilitating comorbid illnesses.

Additional predictors of poor survival after PE include syncope and arterial hypotension. Evidence of right ventricular dysfunction, either clinically, echocardiographically,[13,14] or by plasma markers (e.g., cardiac troponin T, brain natriuretic peptide) predict poor survival among normotensive PE patients.

Recurrent VTE

VTE recurs frequently; about 30 per cent of patients will develop a recurrent episode within the next 10 years (Fig. 2.5).[12,15] The risk of recurrence varies

Table 2.2 Independent predictors of death within 7 days after VTE.[12] Reproduced with permission from *Archives of Internal Medicine* 1999;1598:445–58. Copyright American Medical Association. All rights reserved.

Characteristic	Odds ratio	95 per cent CI
Event year (per increasing year)	0.96	0.94, 0.98
Male sex (among patients with no malignancy)	1.44	1.07, 1.93
BMI (kg/m^2)		
Underweight (BMI < 20)	2.67	1.92, 2.71
Normal weight (20 ≤ BMI < 24)	1.00	—
Overweight (24 < BMI < 30)	0.63	0.46, 0.86
Obese (BMI ≥ 30)	0.56	0.36, 0.86
Location at onset of VTE and age:		
Community:		
45 years old	1.00	—
60 years old	2.05	163, 2.57
75 years old	4.18	2.65, 6.60
Hospital:		
45 years old	13.68	8.07, 23.17
60 years old	17.62	11.00, 29.19
75 years old	23.48	14.33, 38.48
Nursing home:		
45 years old	8.64	2.96, 25.19
60 years old	12.32	5.77, 26.29
75 years old	17.57	10.02, 30.81
Neurologic disease*	1.68	1.16, 2.44
Chronic lung disease*	1.41	1.01, 1.95
Congestive heart failure space assets	2.31	1.72, 3.11
Malignancy without chemotherapy:†		
Female	7.04	4.26, 11.63
Male	2.38	1.47, 3.86
Malignancy with chemotherapy:†		
Female	4.13	2.02, 8.45
Male	8.52	3.76, 19.27
Any surgery and interval between surgery and VTE:		
No surgery in previous 90 days	1.00	—
Surgery within previous 0–21 days	0.36	0.25, 0.51
Surgery within previous 22–90 days	0.71	0.45, 1.12
Hormone therapy *	0.34	2117, 0.71

* The comparison group lacks the indicated characteristic

† Compared to female patients with no malignancy

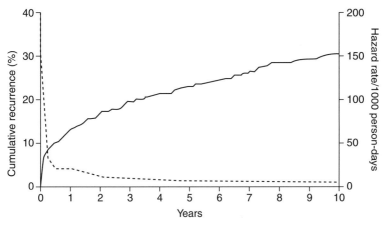

Fig. 2.5 Cumulative incidence of first VTE recurrence (—), and the hazard of first recurrence per 1000 person-days (– – –).[12] Reproduced with permission from *Archives of Internal Medicine* 2000;160:761–8. Copyright American Medical Association. All rights reserved.

with the time since the incident event and is the highest within the first 12 months, but never plateaus off. Even ten years after the incident VTE, patients still are at risk of recurrence. While adequate anticoagulation is effective in reducing the risk of recurrence,[16,17] the duration of anticoagulation does not affect the risk of recurrence once primary therapy for the incident event is stopped.[18–20] Independent predictors of recurrence include male gender,[12] increasing patient age and BMI, neurological disease with extremity paresis, and active malignancy (Tables 2.3 and 2.4).[12,15,21] Additional predictors of recurrence include 'idiopathic' VTE,[17,18,21] lupus anticoagulant or antiphospholipid antibodies,[22] antithrombin, protein C or protein S deficiency,

Table 2.3 Independent predictors of first overall VTE recurrence.[12] Reproduced with permission from *Archives of Internal Medicine* 2000;160:761–8. Copyright American Medical Association. All rights reserved.

Baseline characteristic	Hazard ratio	95 per cent CI
Age*	1.17	1.11, 1.24
BMI†	1.24	1.04, 1.47
Neurological disease with extremity paresis	1.87	1.28, 2.73
Malignancy:		
None	1.00	—
Malignancy with chemotherapy	4.24	2.58, 6.95
Malignancy without chemotherapy	2.21	1.60, 2.06

* per decade increase in age

† per 10 kg/m^2 increase in BMI

Table 2.4 Risk factors for recurrent VTE.

Characteristic	Relative risk
Male gender	1.3–3.6
Age at diagnosis (per decade increase in age)	~1.2
Calf vein thrombosis	~ 0.5
PE versus proximal DVT	1.0
Second VTE	~1.5–2
Antiphospholipid antibody	2.0–4.0
Factor V Leiden heterozygosity	~1.4
Prothrombin G20210A heterozygosity	1.2–1.7
Protein C, protein S, antithrombin deficiency	1–4
Cancer	~3
Elevated D-dimer	~2.4
Residual DVT	1–4
Low thrombin generation potential	0.4
VTE secondary to recent surgery, trauma, or fracture	~0.5

persistent residual DVT, and an elevated D-dimer or increased thrombin generation following the discontinuation of anticoagulation.[23]

Several baseline characteristics that are risk factors for incident VTE are associated with either a reduced risk of recurrence or are not predictive of recurrence. For women, VTE associated with pregnancy or the postpartum state, oral contraceptive use, or gynecologic surgery is associated with reduced risk of recurrence.[12] Recent surgery, trauma, or fracture either have no effect on recurrence[12] or are associated with lower risk of recurrence.[15,21] Recent immobilization, hormone or tamoxifen therapy, and failed prophylaxis have no effect on recurrence rates.[12] The incident VTE event type (i.e., DVT alone versus PE) is not a predictor of recurrence; however, patients with recurrence are significantly more likely to recur with the same event type as the incident event.[24]

Post-thrombotic syndrome

Post-thrombotic syndrome (PTS)—also known as post-phlebitic syndrome or venous stasis syndrome—is a long-term complication of DVT. Owing to the poor long-term prognosis of patients with advanced cancer, PTS is infrequently reported in the palliative care setting, However, it is likely to become an increasing issue within the elderly population and longer-surviving patients with non-malignant disease. The classic symptoms of PTS are dependent swelling and pain of the affected leg, venous ectasia, and skin induration. Severe PTS can lead to painful intractable venous leg ulcers that decrease mobility and require medical and nursing care. Even in less severe cases, the quality of life (QoL) and functional status of affected patients may be impaired.[25,26]

The estimated annual incidence is 76 per 100,000 person-years for venous stasis syndrome and 18 per 100,000 person-years for venous ulcer.[27] Around 30–50 per cent of patients with symptomatic DVT are likely to suffer from PTS within 2 years, and up to 10 per cent will develop venous ulcers within 1–2 years. The cumulative incidence of PTS continues to increase for 20 years following an incident DVT, highlighting the fact that the risk of PTS persists long term.[28]

Venous hypertension and abnormal microcirculation leading to tissue hypoxia have been postulated to be the main predisposing factors for PTS. Venous hypertension results from valvular destruction, venous incompetence, and/or persistent venous outflow obstruction. DVT is usually responsible for venous valve damage, either due to thrombus-induced inflammation or from physical scarring, leading to valvular incompetence.[29] Incomplete vein recanalization following DVT may also obstruct venous outflow leading to collateral circulation via superficial and perforator veins, which gradually become incompetent and varicose.

Chronic thromboembolic pulmonary hypertension

Chronic thromboembolic pulmonary hypertension (CTEPH) occurs rarely in PE patients who fail to completely lyse the thrombus in the pulmonary artery, leading to significant impairment due to chronic shortness of breath and heart failure. Fortunately, this complication is relatively rare affecting only four per cent of all PE patients.[30,31]

Risk factors for VTE

Symptomatic VTE is due to dysregulation of the normal hemostatic response to vessel wall 'injury' that occurs with exposure to a clinical risk factor. However, the vast majority of individuals who are exposed to a clinical risk factor do not develop symptomatic thrombosis. We now recognize that clinical VTE is a multifactorial disease that becomes manifest when a person with an underlying predisposition to thrombosis (i.e., a thrombophilia[s]) is exposed to additional risk factors. Please refer to Tables 2.5 and 2.6 for the list of known acquired and hereditary thrombophilias, and to Table 2.6 for some of the independent risk factors associated with VTE.

Table 2.5 Acquired or secondary thrombophilia.

Strongly supportive data:

- Active malignant neoplasm
- Chemotherapy (L-asparaginase, thalidomide, antiangiogenesis therapy)
- Myeloproliferative disorders
- Heparin-induced thrombocytopenia and thrombosis (HITT)
- Nephrotic syndrome
- Intravascular coagulation and fibrinolysis/disseminated intravascular coagulation (ICF/DIC)
- Thrombotic thrombocytopenic purpura (TTP)
- Sickle cell disease
- Oral contraceptives
- Oestrogen therapy
- Pregnancy/post partum state
- Tamoxifen and raloxifene therapy (selective oestrogen receptor modulator [SERM])
- Antiphospholipid antibodies (lupus anticoagulant, anticardiolipin antibody, antibeta-2 glycoprotein-1 antibody)
- Paroxysmal nocturnal hemoglobinuria (PNH)
- Wegener's granulomatosis

Supportive data:

- Inflammatory bowel disease
- Thromboangiitis obliterans (Buerger's disease)
- Behçet's syndrome
- Varicose veins
- Systemic lupus erythematosus
- Venous vascular anomalies (e.g., Klippel–Trénaunay syndrome)
- Progesterone therapy
- Infertility 'therapy'
- Hyperhomocysteinemia
- HIV infection
- Dehydration

As discussed previously, increasing age is an independent risk factor for the idiopathic and secondary VTE, suggesting that the risk associated with advancing age may be due to biology of aging rather than simply an increased exposure to VTE risk factors with advancing age.[32]

Compared to individuals residing in the community, hospitalized patients have over a 100-fold increased incidence of acute VTE.[3] Hospitalization and nursing home residence together account for almost 60 per cent of all incident VTE events occurring in the community.[32] Of note, hospitalization for medical illness and for surgery account for almost equal proportions of VTE

Table 2.6 Hereditary (familial or primary) thrombophilia.

Strongly supportive data:

- Antithrombin III deficiency
- Protein C deficiency
- Protein S deficiency
- Activated protein C (APC) resistance
- Factor V Leiden
- Prothrombin G20210A
- Homocystinuria

Supportive data:

- Increased plasma factors I (fibrinogen), II (prothrombin), VIII, IX, XI
- Hyperhomocysteinemia
- Dysfibrinogenemia
- Hypoplasminogenemia and dysplasminogenemia
- Hypofibrinolysis
- Reduced protein Z and Z-dependent protease inhibitor (ZPI)
- Reduced tissue factor pathway inhibitor (TFPI)

Weakly supportive data:

- Tissue plasminogen activator (TPA) deficiency
- Increased plasminogen activator inhibitor (PAI-1) levels
- Methylene tetrahydrofolate reductase (MTHFR) polymorphisms
- Factor XIII polymorphisms
- Increased thrombin-activatable fibrinolysis inhibitor (TAFI)

(22 per cent and 24 per cent, respectively). The risk among surgery patients can be further stratified based on patient age, the type of surgery, and the presence of active cancer.[33,34] The incidence of postoperative VTE is increased for surgery patients over 65 years of age. High-risk surgical procedures include major orthopedic surgery of the leg, neurosurgery, thoracic, abdominal, or pelvic surgery for malignancy, renal transplantation, and cardiovascular surgery.[33] After controlling for age, type of surgery, and cancer, additional independent risk factors for incident VTE after major surgery include increasing BMI, intensive care unit confinement for more than 6 days, immobility, infection, and varicose veins.[35] The risk from surgery may be less with neuraxial (spinal or epidural) anesthesia compared to general anesthesia. Independent risk factors for incident VTE among patients hospitalized for acute medical illness include increasing age and BMI, active cancer, neurological disease with extremity paresis, immobility, fracture, and prior superficial vein thrombosis.[36,37]

Table 2.7 Independent risk factors for DVT or PE.[12] Reproduced with permission from *Archives of Internal Medicine* 2000;160:761–8. Copyright American Medical Association. All rights reserved.

Baseline characteristic	Odds ratio	95 per cent CI
Hospitalization:		
Hospitalization for acute medical illness	7.98	4.49, 14.18
Hospitalization for major surgery	21.72	9.44, 49.93
Trauma	12.69	4.06, 39.66
Malignancy without chemotherapy	4.05	1.93, 8.52
Malignancy with chemotherapy	6.53	2.11, 20.23
Prior central venous catheter or transvenous pacemaker	5.55	1.57, 19.58
Prior superficial vein thrombosis	4.32	1.76, 10.61
Neurologic disease with extremity paresis	3.04	1.25, 7.38
Serious liver disease	0.10	0.01, 0.71

Active cancer accounts for almost 20 per cent of incident VTE events occurring in the community.[32] VTE risk among active cancer patients can be further stratified by tumor site, presence of distant metastases, and active chemotherapy. Although all active cancer patients are at risk, the risk appears to be higher for pancreatic cancer, lymphoma, malignant brain tumors, hepatocellular, leukemia, colorectal and other digestive cancers, and for patients with distant metastases.[38–42] Cancer patients receiving cytotoxic, immunomodulating, or antiangiogenic therapy are at even higher risk for VTE[2,39] including chemotherapeutic agents L-asparaginase, cisplatin, 5-fluorouracil, bleomycin, mitomycin, anthracyclines like doxorubicin, immuno-modulators like thalidomide and lenalidomide, other angiogenesis inhibitors like bevacizumab, and hormonal manipulators like tamoxifen and anastrozole (an aromatase inhibitor). In addition, supportive therapy with hematopoetic growth factors like recombinant human erythropoietins and granulocyte-colony stimulating factor (G-CSF) are associated with increased VTE risk.[43]

Central venous catheters or transvenous pacemaker account for about 9 per cent of incident VTE occurring in the community.[31] Prior superficial vein thrombosis is an independent risk factor for subsequent DVT or PE remote from the episode of superficial thrombophlebitis.[2] The risk of DVT imparted by varicose veins is uncertain but appears to be higher among persons less than 40 years of age.[2] Long haul (> 6 hours) air travel is associated with a slightly increased risk for VTE.[44,45] Women receiving therapy with the selective oestrogen receptor modulators tamoxifen and raloxifene also are at increased risk for VTE.

Other conditions associated with VTE include HITT, myeloproliferative disorders (especially polycythemia rubra vera and essential thrombocythemia), ICF/DIC, nephrotic syndrome, paroxysmal nocturnal hemoglobinuria, thromboangiitis obliterans (Buerger's disease), TTP, Behçet's syndrome, systemic lupus erythematosus, Wegener's granulomatosis, inflammatory bowel disease, and homocystinuria.[46] Data for hyperhomocysteinemia is conflicting. Moreover, lowering an elevated homocysteine level in individuals to the normal range with vitamins B6, B12, and folic acid is ineffective for primary or secondary prevention of VTE, thus suggesting that homocysteine may not be playing a direct role in the pathophysiology of VTE.[47] The use of atypical antipsychotic medications, especially in the elderly NH patients appear to increase the risk of VTE.[48]

Genetic risk factors

Recent family-based studies indicate that VTE is highly heritable and follows a complex mode of inheritance involving environmental interaction.[49–51] Inherited reductions in plasma natural anticoagulants (e.g., antithrombin III, protein C, or protein S) have long been recognized as uncommon but potent risk factors for VTE (Table 2.8).[52–54] More recent discoveries of additional reduced natural anticoagulants (e.g., tissue factor pathway inhibitor and protein Z) or anticoagulant cofactors (e.g., fibrinogen gamma-chain), impaired downregulation of the procoagulant system (e.g., activated protein C resistance, factor V Leiden), increased plasma concentrations of procoagulant factors (e.g., factors I [fibrinogen], II [prothrombin], VIII, IX, and XI)[55] and increased basal procoagulant activity, impaired fibrinolysis, and increased basal innate immunity activity and reactivity[56] have added new paradigms to the list of inherited or acquired disorders predisposing to thrombosis (thrombophilia). These plasma hemostasis-related factors or markers of coagulation activation both correlate with increased thrombotic risk and are highly heritable. Inherited thrombophilias interact with such clinical risk factors (e.g., environmental exposures) as oral contraceptives, pregnancy, hormone therapy, surgery and cancer to compound the risk of incident VTE. For example, among female factor V Leiden carriers of peri-menopausal age, the relative risk of VTE associated with hormone therapy may be increased 7- to 15-fold. Similarly, genetic interaction increases the risk of incident VTE. For example, carriers of factor V Leiden mutation with elevated factor VIII or thrombin activatable fibrinolysis inhibitor (TAFI) have a 3-fold higher risk for VTE compared to carriers of factor V Leiden mutation with normal factor VIII and TAFI.[57]

Table 2.8 Familial or acquired thrombophilia: estimated prevalence by population, and incidence and relative risk of incident or recurrent VTE by thrombophilia.

Thrombophilia	Prevalence (whites, per cent)			Incident VTE		Recurrent VTE	
	Normal	Incident VTE	Recurrent VTE	Incidence* (95 per cent CI)	Relative risk (95 per cent CI)	Incidence* (95 per cent CI)	Relative risk (95 per cent CI)
Antithrombin III deficiency	0.02–0.04	1–2	2–5	500 (320, 730)	17.5 (9.1, 33.8)	10,500 (3,800, 23,000)	2.5
Protein C deficiency	0.02–0.05	2–5	5–10	310 (530, 930)	11.3 (5.7, 22.3)	5,100 (2,500, 9400)	2.5
Protein S deficiency	0.01–1	1–3	5–10	710 (530, 930)	32.4 (16.7, 62.9)	6,500 (2,800, 11,800)	2.5
Factor V Leiden†	3–7	12–20	10–50	150 (80, 260)	4.3‡ (1.9, 9.7)	3,500 (1,900, 6100)	1.3 (1.0, 3.3)
Prothrombin G20210A†	1–3	3–8	15–20	350	1.9 (0.9, 4.1)	—	1.4 (0.9, 2.0)
Combined	—	—	—	840 (560, 1220)	32.4 (16.7, 62.9)	5,000 (2,000, 10,300)	—
Antiphospholipid Ab	—	—	—	—	—	—	2.5
Factor VIII (200 IU/dL)	—	—	—	—	—	—	1.8 (1.0, 3.3)

* per 100,000 person-years

† Heterozygous carriers

‡ Homozygous carriers relative risk=80

Data regarding the risk of recurrent VTE among isolated heterozygous carriers for either the factor V Leiden or the prothrombin G20210A mutation are conflicting but the magnitude of increase in the risk is modest. In the meta-analysis by Ho *et al.*,[58] pooled results from ten studies involving 3104 patients with incident VTE revealed that the factor V Leiden mutation was present in 21.4 per cent of patients and associated with a 1.41-fold increased risk for recurrent VTE (95 per cent CI, 1.14–1.75). Similarly, pooled results from nine studies involving 2903 patients revealed that the prothrombin G20210A muta-tion was present in 9.7 per cent and associated with a 1.72-fold increased risk of recurrence (95 per cent CI, 1.27–2.31). The estimated population-attributable risk of recurrence was 9.0 per cent and 6.7 per cent for the factor V Leiden and the prothrombin G20210A mutations, respectively.

Summary

VTE is a common disorder in patients with advanced medical diseases and the elderly population, with significant morbidity and mortality. These groups of individuals have a higher prevalence of environmental/acquired risk factors linked with VTE, especially immobilization—which, in part, accounts for their higher VTE incidence. Moreover, genetic and acquired abnormalities of the coagulation system play a very important role in the pathogenesis of VTE in this population. Reducing its burden in a population with advanced disease will be discussed in later chapters.

References

1. Health, United States, 2006: With Chartbook on Trends in the Health of Americans. 2006 Accessed 6 February 2008; Available from URL:http://www.cdc.gov/nchs/data/hus/hus06.pdf

2. Heit JA, Silverstein MD, Mohr DN *et al*. Risk factors for deep vein thrombosis and pulmonary embolism: a population-based case-control study. *Archives of Internal Medicine* 2000 Mar 27;160(6):809–15.

3. Heit JA, Melton LJ, 3rd, Lohse CM *et al*. Incidence of venous thromboembolism in hospitalized patients vs community residents. *Mayo Clinic proceedings* 2001 Nov; 76(11):1102–10.

4. CMS Data Compendium – 2006 Edition. 2006 [cited 2007 Nov 20]; Available from URL: http://www.cms.hhs.gov/DataCompendium/18_2006_Data_Compendium.asp

5. Jones A. The national nursing home survey: 1999 summary. *Vital and health statistics* 2002 Jun;(152):1–116.

6. Silverstein MD, Heit JA, Mohr DN *et al*. Trends in the incidence of deep vein thrombosis and pulmonary embolism: a 25-year population-based study. *Archives of Internal Medicine* 1998 Mar 23;158(6):585–93.

7. Mehrotra C, Remington PL, Naimi TS *et al*. Trends in total knee replacement surgeries and implications for public health, 1990-2000. *Public Health Reports* 2005 May–Jun; 120(3):278–82.

8. Kobbervig CE, Heit JA, Petterson TM *et al.* The effect of patient age and calendar year on the incidence of idiopathic vs. secondary venous thromboembolism (VTE): a population-based cohort study. *Blood* 2004;104(11):957a (Abstract #3516).

9. White RH, Zhou H, Romano PS. Incidence of idiopathic deep venous thrombosis and secondary thromboembolism among ethnic groups in California. *Annals of Internal Medicine* 1998 May 1;128(9):737–40.

10. White RH, Zhou H, Murin S *et al.* Effect of ethnicity and gender on the incidence of venous thromboembolism in a diverse population in California in 1996. *Thrombosis and Haemostasis* 2005 Feb;93(2):298–305.

11. Heit JA, Cohen AT, Anderson FA, Jr. Estimated annual number of incident and recurrent, non-fatal and fatal venous thromboembolism (VTE) events in the US. *Blood* 2005 November 16;106(11): 267a (Abstract #910).

12. Heit JA, Mohr DN, Silverstein MD *et al.* Predictors of recurrence after deep vein thrombosis and pulmonary embolism: a population-based cohort study. *Archives of Internal Medicine* 2000 Mar 27;160(6):761–8.

13. Goldhaber SZ, Visani L, De Rosa M. Acute pulmonary embolism: clinical outcomes in the International Cooperative Pulmonary Embolism Registry (ICOPER). *Lancet* 1999 Apr 24;353(9162):1386–9.

14. Grifoni S, Olivotto I, Cecchini P *et al.* Short-term clinical outcome of patients with acute pulmonary embolism, normal blood pressure, and echocardiographic right ventricular dysfunction. *Circulation* 2000 Jun 20;101(24):2817–22.

15. Prandoni P, Lensing AW, Cogo A *et al.* The long-term clinical course of acute deep venous thrombosis. *Annals of Internal Medicine* 1996;125(1):1–7.

16. Schulman S, Granqvist S, Holmstrom M *et al.* The duration of oral anticoagulant therapy after a second episode of venous thromboembolism. The Duration of Anticoagulation Trial Study Group [see comments]. *The New England Journal of Medicine* 1997;336(6):393–8.

17. Kearon C, Gent M, Hirsh J *et al.* A comparison of three months of anticoagulation with extended anticoagulation for a first episode of idiopathic venous thromboembolism [published erratum appears in N Engl J Med 1999 Jul 22;341(4):298]. *The New England Journal of Medicine* 1999;340(12):901–7.

18. Agnelli G, Prandoni P, Santamaria MG *et al.* Three months versus one year of oral anticoagulant therapy for idiopathic deep venous thrombosis. Warfarin Optimal Duration Italian Trial Investigators. *The New England Journal of Medicine* 2001;345(3):165–9.

19. Agnelli G, Prandoni P, Becattini C *et al.* Extended oral anticoagulant therapy after a first episode of pulmonary embolism. *Annals of Internal Medicine* 2003 Jul 1;139(1):19–25.

20. Campbell IA, Bentley DP, Prescott RJ *et al.* Anticoagulation for three versus six months in patients with deep vein thrombosis or pulmonary embolism, or both: randomised trial. *British Medical Journal* (Clinical research ed.) 2007 Mar 31;334(7595):674.

21. Baglin T, Luddington R, Brown K *et al.* Incidence of recurrent venous thromboembolism in relation to clinical and thrombophilic risk factors: prospective cohort study. *Lancet* 2003 Aug 16;362(9383):523–6.

22. Schulman S, Svenungsson E, Granqvist S. Anticardiolipin antibodies predict early recurrence of thromboembolism and death among patients with venous thromboembolism following anticoagulant therapy. Duration of Anticoagulation Study Group. *The American Journal of Medicine* 1998 Apr;104(4):332–8.

23. van den Belt AG, Sanson BJ, Simioni P *et al*. Recurrence of venous thromboembolism in patients with familial thrombophilia. *Archives of Internal Medicine* 1997 Oct 27; 157(19):2227–32.

24. Heit JA, S.A. F, Petterson TM *et al*. Venous thromboembolism event type (PE ± DVT vs. DVT) predicts recurrence type and survival. *Blood* 2002;100:149a (Abstract #560).

25. Kahn SR, Hirsch A, Shrier I. Effect of postthrombotic syndrome on health-related quality of life after deep venous thrombosis. *Archives of Internal Medicine* 2002 May 27;162(10):1144–8.

26. Kahn SR, M'Lan CE, Lamping DL *et al*. The influence of venous thromboembolism on quality of life and severity of chronic venous disease. *Journal of Thrombosis and Haemostasis* 2004 Dec;2(12):2146–51.

27. Heit JA, Rooke TW, Silverstein MD *et al*. Trends in the incidence of venous stasis syndrome and venous ulcer: a 25-year population-based study. *Journal of Vascular Surgery* 2001 May;33(5):1022–7.

28. Kahn SR. The post-thrombotic syndrome: the forgotten morbidity of deep venous thrombosis. *Journal of Thrombosis and Thrombolysis* 2006 Feb;21(1):41–8.

29. Bergan JJ, Schmid-Schonbein GW, Smith PD *et al*. Chronic venous disease. *The New England Journal of Medicine* 2006 Aug 3;355(5):488–98.

30. Dunn WF, Heit JA, Farmer SA *et al*. The incidence of chronic thromboembolic pulmonary hypertension (CTEPH): a 25-year population-based study. *European Respiratory Society 13th Annual Congress*. 2003:Abstract P2927.

31. Pengo V, Lensing AW, Prins MH *et al*. Incidence of chronic thromboembolic pulmonary hypertension after pulmonary embolism. *The New England Journal of Medicine* 2004 May 27;350(22):2257–64.

32. Heit JA, O'Fallon WM, Petterson TM *et al*. Relative impact of risk factors for deep vein thrombosis and pulmonary embolism: a population-based study. *Archives of Internal Medicine* 2002 Jun 10;162(11):1245–8.

33. White RH, Zhou H, Romano PS. Incidence of symptomatic venous thromboembolism after different elective or urgent surgical procedures. *Thrombosis and Haemostasis* 2003 Sep;90(3):446–55.

34. Geerts WH, Pineo GF, Heit JA *et al*. Prevention of venous thromboembolism: the Seventh ACCP Conference on Antithrombotic and Thrombolytic Therapy. *Chest* 2004 Sep;126(3 Suppl):338S–400S.

35. White RH, Gettner S, Newman JM *et al*. Predictors of rehospitalization for symptomatic venous thromboembolism after total hip arthroplasty. *The New England Journal of Medicine* 2000 Dec 14;343(24):1758–64.

36. Alikhan R, Cohen AT, Combe S *et al*. Risk factors for venous thromboembolism in hospitalized patients with acute medical illness: analysis of the MEDENOX Study. *Archives of Internal Medicine* 2004 May 10;164(9):963–8.

37. Zakai NA, Wright J, Cushman M. Risk factors for venous thrombosis in medical inpatients: validation of a thrombosis risk score. *Journal of Thrombosis and Haemostasis* 2004 Dec;2(12):2156–61.

38. Heit JA, Petterson TM, Marks RS *et al*. The risk of venous thromboembolism (VTE) among cancer patients by tumor site: a population-based study. *Blood* (ASH Annual Meeting Abstracts) 2004 November 16, 2004;104(11):2596–7.

39. Blom JW, Doggen CJ, Osanto S *et al*. Malignancies, prothrombotic mutations, and the risk of venous thrombosis. *The Journal of the American Medical Association* 2005 Feb 9;293(6):715–22.

40. Blom JW, Vanderschoot JP, Oostindier MJ *et al*. Incidence of venous thrombosis in a large cohort of 66,329 cancer patients: results of a record linkage study. *Journal of Thrombosis and Haemostasis* 2006 Mar;4(3):529–35.

41. Chew HK, Wun T, Harvey D *et al*. Incidence of venous thromboembolism and its effect on survival among patients with common cancers. *Archives of Internal Medicine* 2006 Feb 27;166(4):458–64.

42. Stein PD, Beemath A, Meyers FA *et al*. Incidence of venous thromboembolism in patients hospitalized with cancer. *The American Journal of Medicine* 2006 Jan; 119(1):60–8.

43. Khorana AA, Francis CW, Culakova E *et al*. Risk factors for chemotherapy-associated venous thromboembolism in a prospective observational study. *Cancer* 2005 Dec 15; 104(12):2822–9.

44. Dalen JE. Economy class syndrome: too much flying or too much sitting? *Archives of Internal Medicine* 2003 Dec 8–22;163(22):2674–6.

45. Chee YL, Watson HG. Air travel and thrombosis. *British Journal of Haematology* 2005 Sep;130(5):671–80.

46. Tsai AW, Cushman M, Tsai MY *et al*. Serum homocysteine, thermolabile variant of methylene tetrahydrofolate reductase (MTHFR), and venous thromboembolism: Longitudinal Investigation of Thromboembolism Etiology (LITE). *American Journal of Hematology* 2003 Mar;72(3):192–200.

47. den Heijer M, Willems HP, Blom HJ *et al*. Homocysteine lowering by B vitamins and the secondary prevention of deep vein thrombosis and pulmonary embolism: a randomized, placebo-controlled, double-blind trial. *Blood* 2007 Jan 1;109(1):139–44.

48. Liperoti R, Pedone C, Lapane KL *et al*. Venous thromboembolism among elderly patients treated with atypical and conventional antipsychotic agents. *Archives of Internal Medicine* 2005 Dec 12–26;165(22):2677–82.

49. Souto JC, Almasy L, Borrell M *et al*. Genetic susceptibility to thrombosis and its relationship to physiological risk factors: the GAIT study. Genetic Analysis of Idiopathic Thrombophilia. *American Journal of Human Genetics* 2000 Dec;67(6):1452–9.

50. Larsen TB, Sorensen HT, Skytthe A *et al*. Major genetic susceptibility for venous thromboembolism in men: a study of Danish twins. *Epidemiology* (Cambridge, MA) 2003 May;14(3):328–32.

51. Heit JA, Phelps MA, Ward SA *et al*. Familial segregation of venous thromboembolism. *Journal of Thrombosis and Haemostasis* 2004 May;2(5):731–6.

52. Sanson BJ, Simioni P, Tormene D *et al*. The incidence of venous thromboembolism in asymptomatic carriers of a deficiency of antithrombin, protein C, or protein S: a prospective cohort study. *Blood* 1999 Dec 1;94(11):3702–6.

53. Folsom AR, Aleksic N, Wang L *et al*. Protein C, antithrombin, and venous thromboembolism incidence: a prospective population-based study. *Arteriosclerosis, Thrombosis, and Vascular Biology* 2002 Jun 1;22(6):1018–22.

54. Vossen CY, Walker ID, Svensson P *et al*. Recurrence rate after a first venous thrombosis in patients with familial thrombophilia. *Arteriosclerosis, Thrombosis, and Vascular Biology* 2005 Sep;25(9):1992–7.

55. Koster T, Blann AD, Briet E *et al.* Role of clotting factor VIII in effect of von Willebrand factor on occurrence of deep-vein thrombosis. *Lancet* 1995 Jan 21;345(8943):152–5.

56. Cicala C, Cirino G. Linkage between inflammation and coagulation: an update on the molecular basis of the crosstalk. *Life Sciences* 1998;62(20):1817–24.

57. Libourel EJ, Bank I, Meinardi JR *et al.* Co-segregation of thrombophilic disorders in factor V Leiden carriers; the contributions of factor VIII, factor XI, thrombin activatable fibrinolysis inhibitor and lipoprotein(a) to the absolute risk of venous thromboembolism. *Haematologica* 2002 Oct;87(10):1068–73.

58. Ho WK, Hankey GJ, Quinlan DJ *et al.* Risk of recurrent venous thromboembolism in patients with common thrombophilia: a systematic review. *Archives of Internal Medicine* 2006 Apr 10;166(7):729–36.

Chapter 3

Pathogenesis of venous thromboembolism in cancer

Sarah J. Lewis

Introduction

In the 21st century, the relationship between thrombosis and cancer is well recognized. This knowledge originates from the work of Rudolf Virchow, a professor of anatomic pathology at Berlin University in the 19th century. He observed via his meticulous autopsy recordings that there were three contributing factors (now known as Virchow's triad) resulting in the development of a thrombus:[1]

1. Abnormalities in the vessel wall
2. Abnormalities in the blood components
3. Abnormalities in the blood flow through the vessels

One hundred and fifty years later, the molecular mechanisms associated with various components of his triad are still being researched but the basic pathological principle of the three factors remains as it was years ago. Thrombus itself is made up of fibrin clot and blood constituents including platelets, red cells, and white cells. Venous thrombus has a higher proportion of red cells compared to arterial thrombus, which is predominantly platelets and fibrin. The development of a thrombus is a multifactorial event with many contributing elements—for example, genetic, environmental, lifestyle (e.g., smoking), as well as the underlying disease.

The blood vessel wall

Endothelial cells within the blood vessel wall have a number of protective antithrombotic features to prevent the *in vivo* activation of haemostasis and to ensure smooth blood flow. These include thrombomodulin and heparin sulphate, which both deactivate thrombin. Thrombomodulin also plays a role in the activation of protein C via its interaction with thrombin; nitric oxide, also known as endothelium-derived relaxing factor (EDRF) and prostaglandins both act as vasodilators and modulate platelet activity, as well as fibrinolytic properties via generation of tissue plasminogen activator (TPA).[2]

In patients with malignancy, the blood vessel wall can be directly affected by tumour cells that invade into the endothelium, or secondary to a surgical procedure including the insertion of central venous catheters for administration of treatments including chemotherapy. Both of these can lead to the exposure of tissue factor, which is the catalyst for the initiation of *in vivo* haemostasis.[2]

Tumour cells also have the ability to affect the carefully balanced endothelial surface, expressing P selectin ligands[3] and promoting the expression of adhesion molecules such as intercellular adhesion molecule (ICAM) and vascular cell adhesion molecule (VCAM), which can alter the phenotype of the endothelial cell from an antithrombotic to a prothrombotic state. These topics will be discussed in more detail in the rest of the chapter.

The blood components

It is well known that tumour cells have multiple effects on all the components of the blood including the coagulation system (particularly related to increased fibrinogen, factor VIII (FVIII) and von Willebrand factor (vWF), which will be further described in this chapter, leading to an overall prothrombotic state.[3]

The blood flow

It is also known that blood flow may be impaired due to activation of clotting factors and platelets leading to stasis, as well as venous stasis due to lack of use of the leg muscle pumps in immobile patients, particularly seen postoperatively—blood simply pools in the lower limbs venous system and there is an overall reduction in forward blood flow back to the heart.

In addition, viscosity is a very important factor affecting blood flow. The fibrinogen concentration as well as the level of plasma proteins is a major determinant of this. Raised alpha, beta, and gamma globulins are often seen with malignancy due to the nonspecific host inflammatory response, and may often be a presenting feature of cancer. Raised globulins may also be the presenting feature of myeloma (a plasma cell malignancy) due to the production of a paraprotein by clonal plasma cells. Certain paraproteins, for example, IgM or A, which circulate as a pentamer and a dimer, respectively, are also known to increase viscosity and indeed produce a hyperviscosity syndrome that may be associated with arterial events, e.g., strokes and myocardial infarctions.

Using Virchow's triad as a basis, the pathogenesis of thrombosis in cancer can then be appreciated.

Trousseau and his syndrome

The relationship between thrombosis and cancer was described long ago in 1865 by Trousseau and the combination of the two conditions is still often called Trousseau's syndrome.[4] However, 43 years prior to this, Bouilland had already described three patients with deep vein thrombosis (DVT) and cancer in a paper published in 1823.[5] Since then, cancer has been recognized to be closely linked to both venous and arterial thromboembolism. This link has since been validated by prospective randomized trials concluding there is a significant risk of venous thromboembolism in patients with cancer.[6] This not only affects those with advanced cancer; it may also be the first sign of cancer in asymptomatic patients.

Clinical presentations

There is significant variation in the clinical presentation of the prothrombotic state associated with cancer. Some patients will have little evidence clinically but laboratory tests will show a raised fibrinogen, thrombocytosis, and a short activated partial thromboplastin time (APTT) secondary to raised FVIII levels, all indicating a more thrombotic state. The APTT may also be prolonged due to either the lupus anticoagulant or clotting factor inhibitors, often seen with plasma cell dyscrasias.

The clinical features will vary from overt DVT and pulmonary embolus (PE), a migratory superficial phlebitis, or more unusually arterial thrombosis secondary to cardiac emboli composed of platelet and fibrin vegetations on the mitral or aortic valve (marantic endocarditis).

Venous thromboembolism (VTE) is a frequent complication of cancer and may also be a risk factor in a significant number of patients leading to the development of cancer in the future.[37] Studies have shown that cancer patients make up to 20 per cent of patients presenting with VTE,[6–10] and cancer was diagnosed in a further 5–10 per cent of idiopathic VTE patients over the following 2 years.[11] This is not only intrinsically due to the tumour and the effect it has on the coagulation system, but also due to surgery and subsequent immobility, modern treatment for cancer (chemotherapy and hormonal therapy), central venous catheters for the administration of such treatments, as well as the increasing age of the population. Table 3.1 indicates well-known risk factors for VTE.

Mortality of patients with cancer and VTE is also higher—12 per cent survival vs. 36 per cent survival in age- and sex-matched cancer patients without VTE.[11] This may mean either these patients have a more aggressive form of cancer, or that they are succumbing earlier due to thrombotic complications

Table 3.1 Risk factors and conditions predisposing for VTE.

- History of VTE
- Prolonged immobility
- Prolonged bed rest or lower limb paralysis
- Surgery: especially orthopaedic operations, and major pelvic or abdominal operations
- Trauma: for example, hip fractures and acute spinal injury
- Obesity: BMI > 30
- Major medical illnesses such as acute myocardial infarction, ischaemic stroke, congestive cardiac failure, acute respiratory failure
- Oestrogen use in pharmacological doses: for example, oral contraception pills, hormone replacement therapy
- Cancer: especially metastatic adenocarcinomas
- Age > 40 years
- Acquired hypercoagulable states: lupus anticoagulant and antiphospholipid antibodies, hyperhomocysteinaemia, dysfibrinogenaemia, myeloproliferative disorders such as polycythaemia rubra vera
- Inherited hypercoagulable states (factor V Leiden mutation), protein C deficiency, protein S deficiency, antithrombin deficiency, prothrombin gene mutation

which may be preventable with better prophylaxis.[12] Alongside this runs a 2–6-fold increase in haemorrhagic complications resulting from the treatment of VTE with anticoagulants which must also be considered.[13]

Adenocarcinomas are thought to confer a higher risk of VTE—this was confirmed by a recent study of 537 lung cancer patients.[14] The thrombotic risk in the cancer patients was 20-fold higher than that of the background population, and subgroup analysis showed a 3-fold increase of VTE in adeno-carcinoma patients compared to those with squamous cell carcinoma.[15]

Further studies have conferred a higher risk of VTE with haematological malignancies, followed by lung cancer and GI cancers.[16] Metastatic disease conferred a higher risk again, as did patients with an inherited thrombophilic defect—for example, factor V Leiden, and the prothrombin gene mutation. The reasons for this will be explored in this chapter and an explanation of the effects tumour cells have on coagulation will be given.

Pathogenesis

Tumour cells can multiply, migrate, and develop the ability to adhere and invade the surrounding tissues.[17] The role of the haemostatic system in these processes is well known to be an important one. Inflammatory processes including cancers will lead to a reactive increase in many plasma procoagulants including fibrinogen, FVIII, and vWF. Aside from this, there are many other ways that tumour cells can intrinsically activate the haemostatic system. Procoagulant products of tumour cells have the ability to interact with blood cells including platelets as well as the plasma proteins necessary for haemostasis and fibrinolysis. Some solid tumours will directly invade the blood vessel wall and consequently expose tissue factor (TF) and thus activate coagulation via the TF–factor VIIa (FVIIa) pathway, for example, renal cell carcinoma.[18] Cytokine release from these tumour cells and the acute phase host response will also contribute to the overall procoagulant tendency of the patient with cancer.[19] The differing thrombogenicity of different cancers will also contribute to the varying incidences of VTE with malignancy—for example, adenocarcinoma (especially of the pancreas) has a very strong association with VTE compared to other histological subtypes of cancer.[13] This is likely to be due to the ability of the mucin produced by adenocarcinoma to cause a nonenzymatic activation of factor X, which in turn can activate coagulation *in vivo*. Therefore, the hypercoagulable state is reached via a number of mechanisms:

- Activation of the coagulation system via TF and FVIIa
- Endothelial cell adhesion

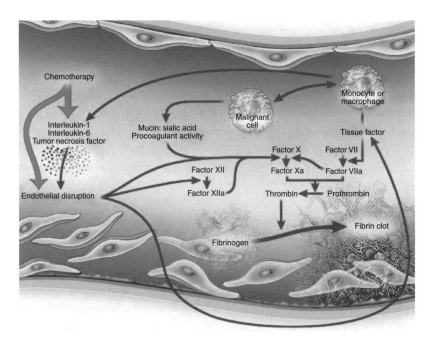

Fig. 3.1 Thrombosis and cancer. Reproduced with permission from Massachusetts Medical Society©. From Bick, RL, *The New England Journal of Medicine* 2003;349: 109–11.

- Inhibition of fibrinolysis via plasminogen activator inhibitor-1 (PAI-1)
- Inhibition of the protein C pathway via the endothelial protein C receptor (EPCR)
- Reduced expression of thrombomodulin via interleukin-1B (IL1B) and tumour necrosis factor (TNF)

TF

This is the initiator of physiological haemostasis *in vivo* and is an integral transmembrane protein usually only found in vascular endothelial cells, neuroglia, vascular smooth muscle, and epidermal cells. It is also expressed by monocytes as well as the endothelium after activation by the inflammatory cytokines, for example, IL6.

The extracellular component of TF acts as both a receptor and a cofactor binding and activating FVII, which, once bound to TF is able as the TF-VIIa complex, to act as the catalyst for thrombin generation via the activation of factor X.[19]

Once thrombin is generated, this leads to fibrin formation and a stable clot. Many types of tumour cells have the ability to express TF on their surface, particularly acute myeloid leukaemia blast cells. Acute promyelocytic leukaemia is well known to cause disseminated intravascular coagulation (DIC) via this pathway—this is characterized by a consumptive coagulopathy leading to severe bleeding due to thrombocytopaenia and reduced clotting factors particularly fibrinogen.

TF expression can also be induced by inflammatory cytokines released by tumour cells, for example TNF and IL1B. These can also up-regulate other proinflammatory molecules, for example, platelet activating factor, PAI-1, and cellular adhesion molecules.[19]

The anticoagulant pathway via activation of protein C via the endothelial cell protein C receptor pathway, and thrombomodulin are both down-regulated by the tumour cells again turning the cell to a procoagulant phenotype.[12]

TF also has an important role in tumour growth. Studies have shown that TF is an important promoter of angiogenesis—TF gene silencing has been shown to inhibit tumour growth as well as tumour spread in research models of TF knockout mice.[21] TF expression in tumour cells is thought to be via the activation of the k-ras oncogene and the loss of the p53 tumour suppressor gene, which would normally play a pivotal role in apoptosis and cell regulation. The proinflammatory cytokines as mentioned earlier (TNF and IL1B) also are pivotal to this process. IL1B and TNF can also directly alter the expression of thrombomodulin and the protein C anticoagulant pathway.[22,35,38]

TF, both alone and complexed with FVIIa, also activates the expression of vascular endothelial growth factor (VEGF),[23] which in turn has a contributing role in angiogenesis, cell adhesion, tumour growth, and tumour spread. It also induces prolonged survival in cells that would normally have undergone apoptosis. TF via the actions of VEGF and other protease activated receptors (PARs) and subsequent cell-signalling mechanisms leading to cell growth and differentiation then tip the balance in favour of a proangiogenic phenotype.[24]

Recent research has shown a direct correlation between TF and oncogenic transformation. Increased levels of TF have been found by Yu *et al.*[21] to be associated with increasing tumour volume as well as increasing oncogenicity of the tumour. Using colorectal cancer cell lines, they also showed that the TF appeared to be concentrated in microparticles within the cell-free supernatant.

TF and thrombin binding have also been shown to enhance urokinase plasminogen activator in prostatic cancer as well as increasing the invasive potential of breast cancer cells.[19,25]

Cancer procoagulant

This is a cysteine protease expressed on tumour cells which has the ability to directly activate FX independent of TF-FVII complexes.[26] This can lead to activation of coagulation as well as increased cell proliferation by its thromboplastin-like action.

Thrombin

The generation of large amounts of thrombin via the TF-VIIa and tenase pathway—known as the thrombin burst—is the central player in physiological haemostasis. It plays a central role in both haemostasis via its action on fibrinogen and subsequent activation of FV, FVIII, FX1, as well as a role in the anticoagulation pathways via TF pathway inhibitor (TFPI), protein C and S, and antithrombin.[27]

Thrombin also enhances expression of TF, VEGF, fibroblast growth factor, via receptors on the cell surface of tumour cells, as well as the vascular endothelium, and subsequently leads to improved cell survival, proliferation, and migration.[27,28]

TF, thrombin, and cancer procoagulant can all activate the coagulation system and this in itself is advantageous for the promotion of tumour cell growth.

The end production of fibrin from fibrinogen is a support structure for angiogenesis as well as protecting against proteolysis. Fibrin has also been shown to be important in cell proliferation and migration via IL-8, a pro angiogenic cytokine.[26,29]

Fibrinolysis

Fibrinolysis usually occurs as a normal haemostatic response to cell injury. TPA released from endothelial cells binds to fibrin and this enhances its capacity to convert clot-bound plasminogen into plasmin. Plasmin then goes on to digest fibrin, fibrinogen, FV, FVIII, releasing fibrin degradation products, for example, fragments X, D, and E. TPA is deactivated by PAI-1, usually preventing widespread digestion of fibrinogen and clotting factors.

Tumour cells have the ability to impair fibrinolysis via actions on many proteins, for example, uPA, tPA, PAI-1, PAI-2 in both promoting and inhibiting manner. This leads to stabilization of the fibrin matrix and subsequent tumour proliferation and spread.[30]

Platelets

Platelets are small granular cytoplasmic fragments derived from megakaryocytes within the bone marrow. They have an important role in primary haemostasis in forming the initial haemostatic plug with vWF. Under high shear conditions circulating platelets can contact exposed subendothelial collagen and adhere to the vessel wall via vWF. This leads to the release of platelet granule contents, which then results in recruitment and aggregation of further platelets. This mechanism leads to the formation of a platelet plug. Along with the presence of calcium ions, exposed phospholipid on the platelet membrane then catalyses the production of FXa and thrombin.

Platelets can also be directly activated by thrombin, and once activated can produce growth factors—VEGF, platelet-derived growth factor (PDGF), which can lead to inhibiting apoptosis and promote angiogenesis again influencing the ability of the tumour to spread.[31]

Tumour cells have the ability to directly activate platelets or to secrete substances known to activate and aggregate platelets, for example, ADP, thrombin, as well as other serine proteases. When activated, platelets can also release their granule contents platelet factor-4 (PF4) and B thromboglobulin. Studies have shown increased levels in patients with active cancers compared to those in remission. These studies also showed increased levels of FVIII and ristocetin cofactor in the platelets as well as reduced sensitivity to prostacyclin.

Platelets, as well as monocytes, endothelial cells, and macrophages, also express P selectin, an adhesion molecule and this can be enhanced by the tumour cells again leading to improved cellular adhesion and migration.[18]

Research has shown that thrombocytopenia has been shown to reduce tumour spread in animal models, an effect that is reversed on correction of the thrombocytopenia.[18]

Platelets have the ability to promote cyclo-oxygenase 2 (COX2) expression in monocytes, and over expression of COX2 can alter the cellular interactions and inhibit cell death, thus producing more invasive tumour behaviour.

Disseminated intravascular coagulation has also been induced recently by Boccaccio *et al* targeting the MET-oncogene in mice.[32] They showed increased PAI-1 and COX 2 expression leading to the development of DIC, suggesting the over expression or mutation of MET oncogene has a significant role to play in the development of intravascular thrombus.[32]

Chemotherapy

Chemotherapy is a well-recognized independent risk factor for VTE, with an annual incidence estimated to be 10–20 per cent.[33,36] Cytotoxic drugs may alter serine protease levels, and also directly damage the endothelium leading to tissue factor exposure and the subsequent activation of the coagulation system.

Hormonal therapies—for example, tamoxifen—may promote thrombosis by reducing natural plasma anticoagulants—for example, protein C and protein S—subsequently promoting the procoagulant phenotype.

Surgery

Surgery is well known to increase the overall prothrombotic tendency as a direct result of TF exposure following traumas to the blood vessels as well as the immobility associated with any operative procedure. Central venous catheters are frequently associated with thrombosis. The thrombogenic surface of the catheter acts as a foreign body within the venous system and will activate platelets as well as FXII and X. Endothelium damage from insertion as well will activate haemostasis in an all-ready at-risk individual with cancer. These catheters are often associated with infections, particularly Gram-negative bacteria that may also lead to produce endotoxins. These sequelae can activate TF, TNF, and interleukins, which will then be able to increase the thrombogenicity of the patient.[33,34]

Venous stasis

This plays an additional role in the multifactorial process of thrombosis. It may be due to bed rest or immobility due to recent surgery or ill health, or due to direct compression on blood vessels by tumour masses or lymph nodes, for example, in the syndrome of superior veno-caval obstruction seen with apical lung tumours or certain lymphomas, particularly those with large mediastinal masses, for example, Hodgkin's disease. The resulting impedance of venous return promotes the development of thrombus along with other contributing factors described by Virchow including an increase in viscosity and coagulation factors as previously described. As the malignant disease progresses and patients spend more time immobile, so too will the anorexia–cachexia syndrome lead to decreased muscle bulk and hence a reduced venous flow via the muscle pump.

All of the above factors become increasingly important as the disease progresses. With the increase in tumour burden, greater procoagulant release is seen via the TF and cancer procoagulant pathways. This subsequently leads to further activation of coagulation and hence the hypercoagulable state. This is compounded by increasing tumour bulk compressing major blood vessels, as well as associated immobility with progressive disease. Metastatic spread leading to bony metastasis can also affect the local microenvironment via inflammatory cytokine release and subsequent activation of coagulation via the mechanisms described above.

Natural anticoagulants

The systemic effects of advanced cancer also need to be considered, for example, anorexia and cachexia, which ultimately lead to hypoalbuminaemia. This will then result in a subsequent decrease in natural anticoagulants (proteins C, S, and antithrombin) which in turn will exacerbate the prothrombotic state further towards the end of life.

Summary

Patients with cancer are more likely to develop VTE than those without. The coagulation cascade is activated by factors related both directly and indirectly to the tumour, and all parts of Virchow's triad may be involved with the development of thrombosis. The degree of the resulting DIC worsens in tandem with the extent of cancer and thus the patient with advanced disease has both a higher risk of VTE and a higher risk of bleeding.

Although ongoing research into the pathogenesis of thrombosis in cancer and the complex interaction between the thrombogenic state and tumour progression is improving our knowledge and understanding, we are left with many unanswered clinical questions in relation to patients with advanced disease such as the optimal management of established VTE, the role of primary thromboprophylaxis, and the possibility of adjuvant anticoagulation as an anticancer therapy.

References

1. Virchow R. *Cellular pathology: as based upon physiological and pathological histology* 1858; Classics of Medicine Library, Birmingham, AL.

2. Greaves M, Lewis SM, Eric P. Pathogenesis of thrombosis and antithrombotic therapy. In Hoffbrand AV, Lewis SM, Tuddenham EGD (eds), *Postgraduate Haematology*, 4e, 1999; Butterworth Heinmann, Oxford, pp. 653–74.

3. Gupta GPMJ. Platelets and metastasis revisited: a novel fatty link. *The Journal of Clinical Investigations* 2004;114:1691–3.

4. Trousseau A. Phlegmasia alba dolens. *Clinical Medicine* (Hotel Dieu Paris) 1865;3:654–712.

5. Bouillard S. De l'obliteration des veines et de son influence sur la formation des hydropisies pateillies consideration sur la hydropisies passive et general. *Archives de médecine générale et tropicale* 2007;1:188–204.

6. Chew HK, Wun T, Harvey D *et al*. Incidence of venous thromboembolism and its effect on survival among patients with common cancers. *Archives of Internal Medicine* 2006;166:458–64.

7. Sorensen HT, Mellemkjaer L, Steffensen FH *et al*. The risk of a diagnosis of cancer after primary deep venous thrombosis or pulmonary embolism. *The New England Journal of Medicine* 1998;338:1169–73.

8. Bick RL. Cancer-associated thrombosis. *The New England Journal of Medicine* 2003;349:109–11.

9. White RH, Chew HK, Zhou H *et al*. Incidence of venous thromboembolism in the year before the diagnosis of cancer in 528,693 adults. *Archives of Internal Medicine* 2005;165:1782–7.

10. Murchison JT, Wylie L, Stockton DL. Excess risk of cancer in patients with primary venous thromboembolism: a national, population-based cohort study. *British Journal of Cancer* 2004;91:92–5.

11. Levitan N, Dowlati A, Remick SC *et al*. Rates of initial and recurrent thromboembolic disease among patients with malignancy versus those without malignancy. Risk analysis using Medicare claims data. *Medicine* 1999;78:285–91.

12. Falanga A, Zacharski L. Deep vein thrombosis in cancer: the scale of the problem and approaches to management. *Annals of Oncology* 2005;16:696–701.

13. Prandoni P, Falanga A, Piccioli A. Cancer and venous thromboembolism. *The Lancet Oncology* 2005;6:401–10.

14. Blom JW, O.S.R FR. The risk of a venous thrombosis is higher with adenocarcinoma than squamous cell carcinoma. *Journal of Thrombosis and Haemostasis* 2007;2:1760–5.

15. Lee AY, Levine MN. Venous thromboembolism and cancer: risks and outcomes. *Circulation* 2003;107:117–21.

16. Blom JW, Doggen CJ, Osanto S *et al*. Malignancies, prothrombotic mutations, and the risk of venous thrombosis. *The Journal of the American Medical Association* 2005; 293:715–22.

17. Bogenrieder T, Herlyn M. Axis of evil: molecular mechanisms of cancer metastasis. *Oncogene* 2003;22:6524–36.

18. Falanga A. Mechanisms of thrombosis in cancer. *Thrombosis Research* 2005; 115(Suppl 1):21–4.

19. Levine MN, Lee AY, Kakkar AK. From Trousseau to targeted therapy: new insights and innovations in thrombosis and cancer. *Journal of Thrombosis and Haemostasis* 2003;1:1456–63.

20. Rosendaal FR. Venous thrombosis: the role of genes, environment and behaviour. *American Society of Haematology Education Book 2005* 2007;1–12.

21. Yu JL, May L, Klement P *et al*. Oncogenes as regulators of tissue factor expression in cancer: implications for tumor angiogenesis and anti-cancer therapy. *Seminars in Thrombosis and Hemostasis* 2004;30:21–30.

22. Grignani G. Cytokines and haemostasis. *Haematologica* 2000;85:967–72.

23. Rao LV, Pendurthi UR. Tissue factor-factor VIIa signaling. *Arteriosclerosis, Thrombosis, and Vascular Biology* 2005;25:47–56.

24. Kwaan HC. The plasminogen-plasmin system in malignancy. *Cancer Metastasis Reviews* 1992;11:291–311.

25. Even-Ram SC, Maoz M, Pokroy E *et al*. Tumor cell invasion is promoted by activation of protease activated receptor-1 in cooperation with the alpha vbeta 5 integrin. *The Journal of Biological Chemistry* 2001;276:10952–62.

26. Rickles FR, Falanga A. Molecular basis for the relationship between thrombosis and cancer. *Thrombosis Research* 2001;102:V215–24.

27. Coughlin SR. Thrombin signalling and protease-activated receptors. *Nature* 2000;407:258–64.

28. Ruf W, Dorfleutner A, Riewald M. Specificity of coagulation factor signalling. *Journal of Thrombosis and Haemostasis* 2003;1:1–495.

29. Qi J, Kreutzer DL. Fibrin activation of vascular endothelial cells. Induction of IL-8 expression. *Journal of Immunology* 1995;155:867–76.

30. Yoshida E, Verrusio EN, Mihara H *et al*. Enhancement of the expression of urokinase-type plasminogen activator from PC-3 human prostate cancer cells by thrombin. *Cancer Research* 1994;54:3300–4.

31. Detmar M. Tumor angiogenesis. *The Journal of Investigative Dermatology* 2000;5:20–3.

32. Boccaccio C, Sabatino G, Medico E *et al*. The MET oncogene drives a genetic programme linking cancer to haemostasis. *Nature* 2005;434:396–400.

33. Baron JA, Gridley G, Weiderpass E *et al*. Venous thromboembolism and cancer. *Lancet* 1998;351:1077–80.

34. Lugassy G, Falanga A, Kakkar A *et al*. Thrombosis and Cancer London: *Martin Dunitz* 2007.

35. Buller HR, Van Doormaal FF, Van Sluis GL *et al*. Cancer and thrombosis: from molecular mechanisms to clinical presentations. *Journal of Thrombosis and Haemostasis* 2007;5:246–54.

36. Otten HM, Prins MH. Venous thromboembolism and occult malignancy. *Thrombosis Research* 2001;102:V187–94.

Chapter 4

Diagnosis of deep vein thrombosis and pulmonary embolism in cancer patients

Menno V. Huisman

Introduction

Cancer is a common cause of venous thromboembolism (VTE) and VTE is a common complication of cancer. Although treatment with anticoagulants is effective, cancer patients still experience a high risk of bleeding and recurrent VTE. Moreover, anticoagulant treatment may compromise and even delay anti-cancer treatment, and this may result in reduced overall survival. Therefore, providing an accurate diagnosis when VTE is suspected in patients with cancer is very important in order to avoid misdiagnosis and inappropriate anticoagulation. This chapter will discuss the diagnostic tools available and outline diagnostic approaches in the following clinical scenarios in patients with cancer: clinically suspected deep vein thrombosis (DVT) of the leg, clinically suspected pulmonary embolism (PE) and clinically suspected upper extremity DVT.

Tests for DVT diagnosis

It is important to appreciate the natural history of DVT when discussing the accuracy and utility of available diagnostic tests. DVT usually starts in the calf or distal veins.[1–3] Approximately 20 per cent will propagate into the popliteal or more proximal veins within a week of the initial presenting symptoms, while the remainder will undergo lysis spontaneously without antithrombotic treatment.[3–5] When DVT causes symptoms, more than 80 per cent of them involve the popliteal or more proximal veins.[2,6] Moreover, non-extending distal DVT rarely causes PE, whereas proximal DVT often does.[7,8] Thus, isolated distal DVT is uncommon in symptomatic patients, isolated non-extending distal DVT is of minor clinical importance, and proximal extension of distal DVT more than a week after presentation is unusual.

Clinical prediction rules

The clinical presentation of DVT is non-specific, but it is helpful for risk stratification. A clinical prediction rule (Wells' rule) that integrates the assessment of signs, symptoms, and risk factors has been validated and is widely used to categorize patients as having a low, moderate, or high probability for DVT (Table 4.1).[9] Based on numerous studies, patients in these risk categories have a prevalence of DVT of approximately 5, 15, and 50 per cent, respectively. More recently, the Wells' rule has been simplified to dichotomize patients into 'DVT likely' or 'DVT unlikely' groups.[10,11] Inter-observer reliability has not been thoroughly studied, but the Wells' rule performs consistently well in different studies involving many different types of physicians with a wide range of clinical experiences. It has been demonstrated that DVT can be safely excluded in patients with a low pre-test probability and a single normal ultrasound test, without the need for serial testing.[12] The prediction rule can also be used in combination with a D-dimer test.

If a patient with cancer develops symptoms suggestive of DVT, the Wells' clinical prediction rule can be applied as a first screening tool. However, the Wells' rule was not developed specifically for cancer patients and the evidence for applying this tool to this population is limited. Cancer patients are more likely to score a moderate or high probability because active malignancy or cancer

Table 4.1 Wells' rule for DVT diagnosis. Reproduced with permission from the International Society on Thrombosis and Haemostasis©. From Wells PS. Integrated strategies for the diagnosis of venous thromboembolism. *Journal of Thrombosis and Haemostasis* 2007;5:41–50.

Clinical variable	Score
Active cancer (treatment ongoing or within previous 6 months or palliative)	1
Paralysis, paresis, or recent plaster immobilization of the lower extremities	1
Recently bedridden for 3 days or more, or major surgery within the previous 12 weeks requiring general or regional anesthesia	1
Localized tenderness along the distribution of the deep venous system	1
Entire leg swelling	1
Calf swelling at least 3 cm larger than that on the asymptomatic leg (measure 10 cm below the tibial tuberosity)	1
Pitting edema confined to the symptomatic leg	1
Collateral superficial veins (non-varicose)	1
Previously documented DVT	1
Alternative diagnosis at least as likely as DVT	−2

DVT, deep vein thrombosis. * ≥2, probability of DVT is 'likely'. ≤1, probability for DVT is 'unlikely'. Alternatively, < 1 is low probability, moderate is 1 or 2, and high is >2.

treatment within the last 6 months is scored with 1 point. Furthermore, because comorbidities in cancer patients and cancer-related factors—such as the stage or extent of malignancy—are not accounted for in the Wells' rule, it is important to keep these in mind when assessing the pre-test probability in these patients.

Contrast venography

Contrast venography is the gold standard for the diagnosis of DVT. Only 0.6 per cent of those with a negative venogram develop a DVT over the next 3 months.[13] However, the method is not ideal because of its invasive nature, its technical demands, the cost, and the risks associated with contrast media. Therefore, several alternative diagnostic methods have been developed, including impedance plethysmography[4,5] and venous ultrasonography (compression ultrasonography with or without Doppler flow assessment).[14,15] Only compression ultrasonography is still widely used and can be considered the non-invasive reference method of choice.

Compression ultrasonography

The technique of compression ultrasonography combines real-time ultrasound imaging and external compression of a venous segment using the ultrasound probe. By using brightness modulation (B-mode) ultrasonography, a two-dimensional image is produced of the cross section of a vessel. If gentle external pressure applied with the ultrasound probe fails to fully compress the cross-sectional diameter of the vein, then intraluminal thrombus is diagnosed. Conversely, the ability to fully compress the lumen of a venous segment excludes DVT.[14,16] Typically, scanning and compression are applied to the common femoral vein, superficial vein, popliteal vein, and the calf trifurcation. Ultrasonography of the calf veins is less reliable and is not routinely performed.

To further evaluate the presence of blood flow around the thrombus, or if the venous segment is not accessible for compression, Doppler techniques that allow the measurement of the direction and speed of blood flow are available. The combination of B-mode imaging and Doppler flow assessment is known as duplex ultrasonography. Display of the Doppler signal as a color image superimposed on the B-mode image is called color Doppler ultrasonography. Although they are widely used, Doppler assessment of blood flow and other B-mode criteria, such as the presence of intraluminal echoes, have not been shown to improve the diagnostic accuracy of compression ultrasonography.

D-dimer testing

D-dimer is a degradation product of cross-linked fibrin. It is typically elevated in patients with acute VTE. D-dimer levels may also be increased by a variety of non-thrombotic disorders, including recent major surgery, hemorrhage, trauma, malignancy, or sepsis. Increasing age and pregnancy are also associated with higher levels of D-dimer.[17,18] Consequently, D-dimer assays are sensitive but non-specific markers for VTE, such that positive D-dimer results are not useful to 'rule in' the diagnosis but a negative result is useful to 'rule out' the diagnosis. Since the sensitivity of various D-dimer assays is approximately 90 to 95 per cent and the specificity is only 55 per cent, the test is well suited for ruling out DVT. However, D-dimer testing cannot be used as the sole test to exclude DVT, because 5 to 10 per cent of DVTs will be missed. Therefore, the test should be used as an adjunct to other diagnostic methods. It is also important to keep in mind that the relatively low specificity of D-dimer testing will produce a high number of false positive results, especially when highly sensitive D-dimer assays are used.

Although it is well documented that the D-dimer test is useful in the diagnostic workup of patients with suspected DVT, this test is less useful in patients with underlying cancer, particularly so in patients with extensive disease. Since D-dimer levels are likely to be elevated in cancer patients even in the absence of thrombosis,[19,20] more patients will have an abnormal and a false positive result.

In a prospective study, the clinical utility of a whole blood D-dimer test (SimpliRed®, Agen Inc., Australia) in patients suspected of having DVT was evaluated.[21] All patients underwent compression ultrasonography of the proximal veins and D-dimer testing on the day of referral. If the D-dimer and ultrasonography results were normal, the patient was considered not to have DVT and no further testing was performed. If the ultrasonography result was normal and the D-dimer test result abnormal, ultrasonography was performed again 1 week later. If this second ultrasonogram result was also normal, DVT was again ruled out. Anticoagulant therapy was only instituted in those patients with an abnormal ultrasound result. All patients were followed up for 3 months to record possible subsequent thromboembolic events. In 63 (29 per cent) of the 217 cancer patients, the D-dimer and ultrasonography results were normal on the day of referral; DVT was considered to be excluded and anticoagulant therapy was withheld. In these 63 patients, one thromboembolic event occurred during follow-up (1.6 per cent; 95 per cent CI, 0.04–8.5 per cent). Therefore, using the D-dimer test, the need for an additional ultrasonogram can potentially be avoided in 29 per cent (95 per cent CI, 23–35 per cent) of the cancer patients with clinically suspected DVT. In a comparative group of non-cancer patients, 0.7 per cent (95 per cent CI, 0.4–1.9 per cent) of patients developed VTE during the 3 months of follow-up, with 50 per cent (95 per cent CI, 48–53 per cent) of the patients not having to undergo further testing.

These encouraging findings are somewhat inconsistent with the results of another study.[22] The negative predictive value of the SimpliRed® D-dimer test in the cohort of 121 cancer patients was significantly lower than in the non-cancer patient group, with values of 79 per cent (95 per cent CI, 63–90 per cent) and 97 per cent (95 per cent CI, 95–98 per cent), respectively. The authors explained this difference was a consequence of the low sensitivity of the D-dimer test (86 per cent) and the higher prevalence of DVT among cancer patients. They concluded that the SimpliRed® D-dimer test is insufficient for accurate DVT diagnosis in cancer patients when used alone.

Another study explored the safety of using the SimpliRed® D-dimer test with a clinical prediction rule for excluding DVT in cancer patients.[23] In this study, it was reported that the negative predictive value of the D-dimer test was 100 per cent (95 per cent CI, 85–100 per cent) and 97 per cent (95 per cent CI, 88–99 per cent) among cancer patients with low or low–moderate probability, respectively. Of note, only 17 per cent of the cancer patients were considered to have a low pre-test probability of DVT, even though 41 per cent had DVT diagnosed.

Overall, there is some evidence that in cancer patients with clinically suspected DVT, a negative D-dimer result might be useful in excluding the diagnosis in the small number of patients with a low or low–moderate pre-test probability. However, larger studies are needed to confirm these findings particularly in patients with advanced disease. Quantitative D-dimer tests with high sensitivity (e.g., Tina-quant® D-dimer, Roche Diagnostics, US; VIDAS® D-dimer, bioMérieux, US) are more suitable for excluding DVT in patients with cancer than D-dimer assays with lower sensitivity, but sensitive assays will produce more false positive results.[24]

Tests for PE diagnosis

It has long been recognized that the diagnosis of PE based on a patient's history and physical examination is non-unspecific. Various clinical prediction rules and diagnostic algorithms have been developed to streamline management and improve accuracy.

Clinical prediction rules

Clinical prediction rules have been developed over the past ten years to help diagnose PE. These rules integrate signs, symptoms, and risk factors, sometimes in combination with electrocardiography (ECG) and chest X-ray results. The most widely used and validated clinical prediction rules are the Wells' rule[25,26] and the Geneva score (Tables 4.2 and 4.3).[27] However, both

Table 4.2 Wells' score for PE diagnosis.[25,26]

Variable	Points
Clinical signs and symptoms of DVT (minimum of leg swelling and pain with palpation of the deep veins)	3
An alternative diagnosis is less likely than PE	3
Heart rate greater than 100	1.5
Immobilization or surgery in the previous 4 weeks	1.5
Previous DVT/PE	1.5
Hemoptysis	1
Malignancy (on treatment, treated in the last 6 months or palliative)	1
Clinical probability	
Low	<2 total
Intermediate	2–6 total
High	>6 total
Dichotomized assessment	
Less likely	≤4 total
Likely	>4 total

scores have limitations. The Wells' rule includes the physician's judgment of whether an alternative diagnosis is more likely than a diagnosis of PE. This criterion carries a major weight in the scoring and cannot be standardized because it is subjective. The Geneva score, based on 13 objective variables, requires a room air blood gas analysis and has only been evaluated in patients in the emergency ward. Both scores appeared to have comparable predictive values for PE, which is 3.6 per cent and 9.0 per cent in the low, 20.5 per cent and 33 per cent in the intermediate, and 66.7 per cent and 66 per cent in the high clinical probability cohorts, respectively. The revised Geneva score is a simplified version that is based on clinical variables, does not require a blood gas analysis, and is independent from physicians' gestalt judgment.[28] Prevalence of PE using the revised Geneva score is 9.0 per cent in the low, 28 per cent in the intermediate, and 72 per cent in the high clinical probability group. Very recently, it was shown that the performance of the revised Geneva score is potentially equivalent to that of the Wells' rule.[29]

Like clinical prediction rules for DVT diagnosis, rules for PE diagnosis also have had limited assessment in patients with cancer. In patients with pulmonary pathology due to their malignancy, for example, malignant effusion, it is particularly difficult to apply these rules because respiratory symptoms are virtually identical in patients with PE and without PE. Similarly, in patients with advanced non-malignant disease, such as heart failure or pulmonary disease, the clinical symptoms of PE may be difficult to distinguish

Table 4.3 Geneva score for PE diagnosis. Reproduced with permission from Wicki J, Perneger TV, Junod AF *et al. Archives of Internal Medicine* 2001;161(1):92–7.

Variable	Points
Age 60–79 years	1
Age >79 years	2
Previous DVT or PE	2
Recent surgery	3
Pulse rate >100/min	1
$PaCO_2$ <4.8 kPa	2
$PaCO_2$ 4.8–5.19 kPa	1
PaO_2 <6.5 kPa	4
PaO_2 6.5–7.99 kPa	3
PaO_2 8–9.49 kPa	2
PaO_2 9.5–10.99 kPa	1
Chest X-ray platelike atelectasis	1
Chet X-ray elevation of hemidiaphragm	1
Clinical probability	
Low	0–4 total
Intermediate	5–8 total
High	>8 total

from those of their underlying illness. Hence, it is important to keep a high index of suspicion in patients with advanced disease and obtain objective testing when the pre-test clinical probability is less certain.

Pulmonary angiography

Pulmonary angiography is regarded as the gold standard test for the diagnosis of PE. Although the procedure is usually well tolerated, it is invasive, expensive, and requires a skilled radiologist and a cooperative patient.[30,31] It is contraindicated in patients with significant pulmonary hypertension and in those with renal insufficiency. In addition, a negative result does not entirely exclude VTE. In the Prospective Investigation of Pulmonary Embolism Diagnosis (PIOPED) study, 1.6 per cent of patients with normal angiograms in developed PE over the 1-year follow-up period, with most of the events occurring in the first month.[32,33]

Ventilation-perfusion lung scan

Ventilation and perfusion (V/Q) lung scanning (Fig. 4.1) was introduced as a non-invasive test with minimal complications. For decades, this method was the imaging procedure of choice in patients with suspected PE and it remains the safest alternative in patients with renal insufficiency. A normal scan essentially excludes the diagnosis of PE (1 per cent VTE rate in follow-up), and a high-probability lung scan has an 85 to 90 per cent positive predictive value

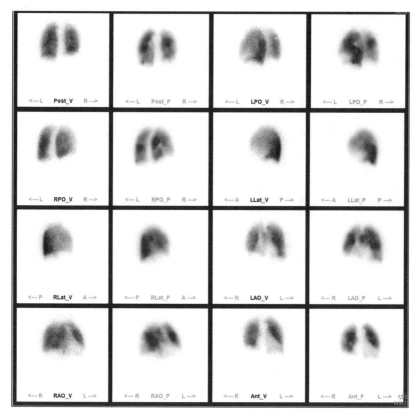

Fig. 4.1 A V/Q scan showing a large segmental filling defect in the anterior aspect of the right middle lobe. There is also a smaller, subsegmental perfusion defect posteriorly within in the right lower lobe and a wedge-shaped area of perfusion defect in the superior segment of the left lower lobe. Ventilation in these areas is normal.

for PE.[32–34] Unfortunately, scans are considered non-diagnostic in 50 to 75 per cent of patients, in which the prevalence of PE varies from 10 to 30 per cent. Non-diagnostic scans are particularly frequent in patients with comorbid lung conditions or abnormal chest X-ray findings, conditions that are common in patients with advanced disease. It is also not widely available because of the need for radioisotopes.

Computed tomographic pulmonary angiography

Single detector contrast computed tomographic pulmonary angiography (CTPA) (Fig. 4.2) became available as a diagnostic test for PE in the early 1990s and multi-row detectors are now common in most hospitals, allowing faster

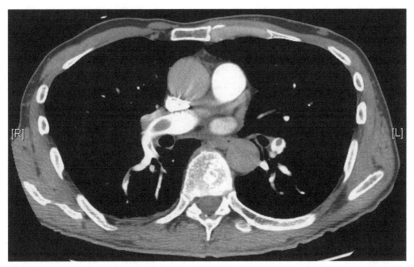

Fig. 4.2 CTPA showing a large intraluminal filling defect is seen in the right main pulmonary artery, extending into the lobar and segmental branches. There is also a smaller filling defect in the left main pulmonary artery.

testing and producing images with higher resolution. CT scanning is more rapidly and widely available than V/Q scanning and CTPA has become the imaging test of choice in many centres. In addition, CTPA provides an alternative diagnosis for presenting symptoms in 25 per cent of the cases. This is particularly useful in patients with advanced disease, as it can not only help the clinician assess the presence or absence of PE, but also other conditions that can contribute to the symptoms. However, CTPA is associated with considerable radiation and iodinated contrast exposure and is contraindicated in patients with renal insufficiency.

In a recent meta-analysis, the pooled sensitivity and the specificity of CTPA were 86 and 94 per cent, respectively.[35] The recently published PIOPED II study[36] reported an excellent specificity of 96 per cent and a sensitivity of 83 per cent for CTPA in the diagnosis of PE with multi-detector CT. Management studies and a randomized clinical trial have shown that CTPA is as good as V/Q scanning for ruling out PE, thus alleviating the initial fears that CT would miss clinically significant PE.[37,38]

Magnetic resonance angiography

The advantages of non-invasiveness and non-ionizing radiation requirement make magnetic resonance (MR) a promising imaging modality for diagnosing PE.

Possible useful techniques in the diagnostic work-up of patients with suspected PE include MR angiography (MRA), thrombus imaging for direct clot visualization, perfusion MR, and combined perfusion-ventilation MR.[39] Although MR imaging was once considered a safe alternative for patients with renal insufficiency, in whom iodinated contrast for CTPA is contraindicated, it is now recognized that such patients are at high risk of developing gadolinium-induced nephrogenic systemic fibrosis (NSF).[40] This is a devastating fibrosing disorder of the skin and other systemic organs, characterized by long-term gadolinium deposits in tissues. Consequently, gadolinium is contraindicated in patients with renal dysfunction.

In a prospective study, in which MRA was compared with conventional pulmonary angiography, a sensitivity of 77 per cent (95 per cent CI, 61–90 per cent), a specificity of 98 per cent (95 per cent CI, 92–100 per cent), a positive predictive value of 93 per cent (95 per cent CI, 78–99 per cent), and negative predictive value of 91 per cent (95 per cent CI, 85–96 per cent) for PE were observed.[41] The safety of withholding anticoagulant treatment in patients with a normal MRA has not been studied. Given the limited data, it is not yet possible to use MRA in a routine patient setting.

Diagnostic management in patients with clinically suspected DVT

In patients with leg symptoms suggestive of DVT initially, the clinical probability should be determined using an established prediction rule such as the Wells' rule. In patients with a low or unlikely pre-test probability, a D-dimer test should be performed. In these patients, a normal D-dimer result can reliably exclude DVT without the need for ultrasonography. Using this strategy, ultrasonography is unnecessary in up to 40 per cent of patients referred with suspected DVT. However, ultrasonography may provide information helpful to establish an alternative diagnosis. More sensitive D-dimer tests, such as the VIDAS® D-dimer test or Tina-quant® test, may be able to reduce the need for ultrasonography in patients with moderate pre-test probability.[24]

All patients with a moderate or high clinical probability or a low probability with a positive D-dimer result should undergo compression ultrasonography. If ultrasound imaging is not readily available, then the patients with moderate or high clinical probability may receive an injection of low molecular weight heparin (LMWH) (treatment dose) while imaging is arranged the following day.[42]

If the ultrasound is positive (lack of complete vein compressibility), the diagnosis of DVT is confirmed. If the ultrasound is negative, then a repeat ultrasound no more then 1 week later is generally recommended. Several studies have reported that in patients with a normal D-dimer result and a normal initial ultrasound, it is safe to exclude DVT without a serial ultrasound test.[42–44] This strategy was validated in at least one study.[43] For patients in the palliative setting, avoiding serial ultrasound testing is also desirable, but it is important to note that false normal D-dimer results may occur in patients with prolonged symptoms of DVT or after prolonged heparin therapy (more than 24 h).

Recommended diagnostic strategies in patients with cancer and suspected DVT

In patients with cancer and clinically suspected DVT, the same strategies can be applied as for patients without cancer, but the role of D-dimer testing is less certain (Figs. 4.3 and 4.4).

As discussed earlier, the SimpliRed test is insufficient to be used as a sole bedside test for cancer patients, and sensitive quantitative D-dimer tests have not been evaluated in this population. The sensitivity of a combination of low clinical probability and normal qualitative D-dimer test was reported as high in one study, but up to 15 per cent of patients with DVT may be missed because the lower bound of the confidence interval was low at 85 per cent. The efficiency of excluding DVT on the basis of a normal ultrasound and normal D-dimer test is also much lower than in patients without cancer because initial and serial ultrasound testing can only be omitted in a small proportion

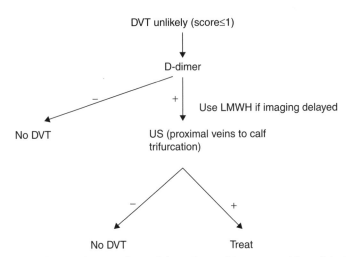

Fig. 4.3 Flow diagram for DVT diagnosis in patients with cancer and low clinical probability. US, ultrasound. Reproduced with permission from the International Society on Thrombosis and Haemostasis©. From Wells PS. Integrated strategies for the diagnosis of venous thromboembolism. *Journal of Thrombosis and Haemostasis* 2007;5:41–50.

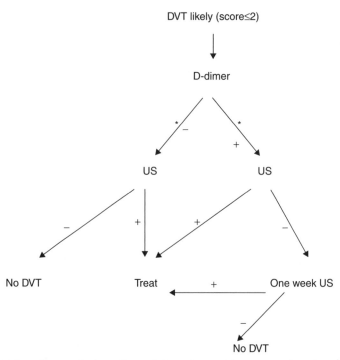

Fig. 4.4 Flow diagram for DVT diagnosis in patients with cancer and moderate/high clinical probability.* use LMWH if imaging is going to be delayed. Reproduced with permission from the International Society on Thrombosis and Haemostasis©. From Wells PS. Integrated strategies for the diagnosis of venous thromboembolism. *Journal of Thrombosis and Haemostasis* 2007;5:41–50.

of patients. According to one study, the three-month VTE failure rate in cancer patients with a normal ultrasound and normal qualitative D-dimer test may be as high as 8.5 per cent.

Overall, it is recommended that all cancer patients undergo pre-test probability assessment, followed by D-dimer test and ultrasonography.

If a patient has a low clinical probability, a D-dimer should initially be performed. If this test is negative, then DVT is excluded. If it is abnormal, an ultrasound should be performed. If this ultrasound is negative, then DVT is excluded. If the ultrasound is abnormal for popliteal or more proximal veins, then the patient has a DVT and should be treated.

If the clinical probability is moderate or high, then ultrasonography should be arranged irrespective of the result of the D-dimer test. If the initial ultrasound is negative and the D-dimer is negative, then DVT is excluded. If the initial ultrasound is negative and the D-dimer test is positive, then a repeat ultrasound should be arranged within the next 7 days (see Figs. 4.3 and 4.4).

Diagnostic management in patients with clinically suspected PE

Patients with suspected PE should initially have an assessment of pre-test probability using an established clinical prediction rule. Three large studies totalling over 4,600 patients have demonstrated that the strategy combining clinical probability, D-dimer tests, and CTPA can safely exclude PE at initial presentation, without the need for further diagnostic imaging.[37,45,46] The Christopher study showed that it is safe to exclude PE and consequently withhold anticoagulant therapy in patients with a less likely clinical probability and a normal D-dimer result or in patients who have a normal CT scan, regardless of their clinical probability for PE or D-dimer result.[37] In this study, 3,305 consecutive patients with suspected PE were included. The clinical probability of PE was prospectively assessed using the Wells' rule. In all patients with a score of 4 or less (less likely diagnosis), a quantitative D-dimer test was performed. In patients with a less likely probability and a normal quantitative D-dimer result, PE was considered excluded. CTPA was performed in patients with a score greater than 4 points or an abnormal quantitative D-dimer result. All patients were followed up for 3 months to evaluate the occurrence of PE. Of the 1,057 patients with a less likely probability and a normal D-dimer result, 29 patients (2.7 per cent) were treated with oral anticoagulants during follow-up for various reasons other than VTE. Three of the 1,028 remaining patients returned with symptomatic VTE events (two nonfatal PE, one DVT) during the 3-month follow-up period, for a VTE failure rate of 0.5 per cent (95 per cent CI, 0.2–1 per cent). Of the 1,505 patients in whom CTPA was negative for PE, 69 (4.6 per cent) received anticoagulants during follow-up for various reasons other than VTE. Of the 1,436 patients who did not receive anticoagulant treatment, 18 experienced VTE events during the 3-month follow-up (1.3 per cent; 95 per cent CI, 0.7–2.0 per cent). Eleven of these patients had non-fatal symptomatic thromboembolic events (three PE and eight DVT). Fatal PE was judged to have occurred in seven patients (0.5 per cent, 95 per cent CI 0.2 to 1.0 per cent). This latter figure is comparable to the 0.8 per cent 3-month fatal PE rate after a normal pulmonary angiography.[32,33]

Based on the Christopher study, the diagnostic strategy of choice in patients with suspected PE starts with an assessment of patients' pre-test probability using the Wells' clinical decision rule. If an unlikely diagnosis of PE is observed, a quantitative D-dimer test with high sensitivity should be performed. In case of a normal D-dimer result, PE can safely be excluded from the differential diagnosis (Fig. 4.5). If the D-dimer is elevated, or if the pre-test probability

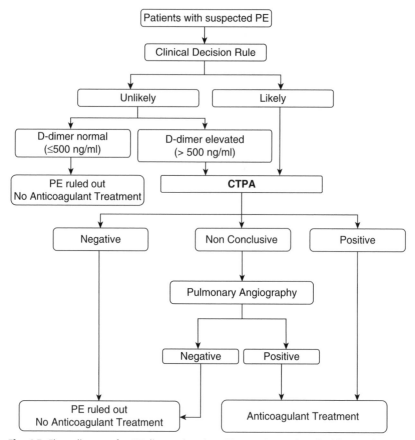

Fig. 4.5 Flow diagram for PE diagnosis using CT scan. Reproduced with permission from Blackwell Publishing©. Karami Djurabi R, Klok FA, Nijkeuter M et al. Integrated diagnostic approach of patients with suspected pulmonary embolism. *Imaging Decisions MRI* 2007;11(3):29–33.

indicates a likely probability of PE, additional diagnostic imaging with either CTPA or V/Q scanning is required. These imaging techniques appear comparable in detecting clinically significant PE.[42] If they are not conclusive, conventional pulmonary angiography is recommended. In patients with leg symptoms, it is reasonable to perform an ultrasound of the leg veins, especially if there were concerns regarding contrast or radiation exposure.

Recommended diagnostic strategies in patients with cancer and suspected PE

Several studies evaluating diagnostic strategies in patients presenting with clinically suspected PE have published the results of the subgroup of patients with cancer. In the first study, the accuracy of a quantitative D-dimer test

(Tina-quant® D-dimer) was assessed in 519 consecutive inpatients and outpatients with clinically suspected PE.[47] All patients were followed-up for 3 months and PE was confirmed based on positive results on radiological imaging. In the 72 cancer patients, the sensitivity and negative predictive value of the D-dimer test were 100 percent, but the 95 per cent CIs were wide and ranged from 82 to 100 percent and 72 to 100 per cent, respectively. The specificity of the D-dimer test was only 21 per cent in patients with cancer. It was concluded from this study that a normal quantitative D-dimer result may safely exclude the diagnosis of PE in patients with cancer.

In a retrospective study, Righini et al. analyzed the usefulness of a quantitative ELISA D-dimer test (VIDAS® D-dimer) in 164 patients with cancer from two separate prospective studies.[48] PE was ruled out by a normal D-dimer and low to intermediate clinical probability, as assessed by the Geneva score, in 32 per cent patients (494 of 1,554) without cancer and in 11 per cent (18 of 164) patients with cancer. The 3-month thromboembolic risk was 0 per cent in cancer patients with a normal D-dimer result and low to intermediate clinical probability, but the upper bound of the confidence limit was 18 per cent.

Finally, in a retrospective analysis of the Christopher study, 479 patients with cancer, who comprised 14 per cent of the total Christopher cohort, were studied.[49] Of these patients, only 49 (10 per cent) had a combination of an unlikely clinical score and normal quantitative D-dimer test, compared with 32 per cent in the total study population. During 3 months of follow-up, one patient (2 per cent; 95 per cent CI, 0.05–10.9 per cent) in this group returned with VTE. In addition, among the 268 cancer patients with likely probability of PE and/or an abnormal D-dimer test, PE was excluded by the initial CT scan; of these patients, five returned with recurrent VTE for a failure rate of 1.8 per cent (95 per cent CI, 0.6–4.0 per cent) for CTPA. This estimate is comparable to the 1.3 per cent in the total Christopher patient group, but the confidence interval is wider.

Based on the evidence to date, the same diagnostic strategy for clinically suspected PE could be applied in patients with or without cancer (Figs. 4.5 and 4.6). However, it is important to note that the efficiency of an unlikely clinical probability and normal D-dimer test is lower in cancer than in non-cancer patients, such that only around 10 per cent of cancer patients will have PE excluded. The majority of 90 per cent patients still need additional imaging. Furthermore, up to 10 per cent of patients with an initially unlikely probability and normal D-dimer result will develop VTE within the next 3 months of follow-up. The diagnosis of PE cannot be excluded on the basis of a D-dimer test alone because the sensitivity (82 per cent) and negative predictive value (72 per cent) are not sufficiently high enough. If the CTPA scan is

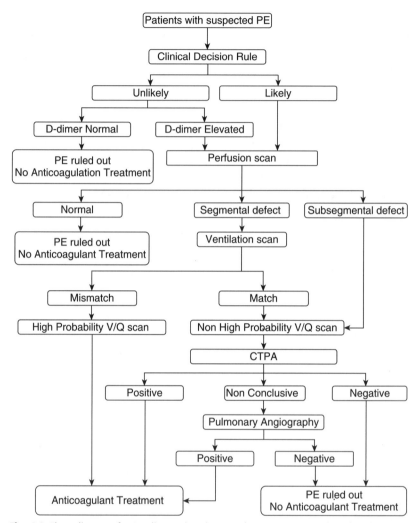

Fig. 4.6 Flow diagram for PE diagnosis using V/Q lung scan. Reproduced with permission from Blackwell Publishing©. Karami Djurabi R, Klok FA, Nijkeuter M *et al*. Integrated diagnostic approach of patients with suspected pulmonary embolism. *Imaging Decisions MRI* 2007;11(3):29–33

negative for PE, up to 4 per cent of patients may present with VTE during the next 3 months of follow-up.

CTPA is costly and involves significant radiation; therefore it could be worth it if D-dimer estimation excluded PE in only 10 per cent of cancer patients. However, the overall experience and validation of diagnostic tests for PE remain limited in cancer patients. Although the published data suggest that normal results are helpful and lower the likelihood of PE, the risk estimates are not well established. Also, cancer patients enrolled in clinical trials may not be representative of the general oncology population. Hence, it remains prudent to maintain a high index of suspicion for PE in this high risk population and perform objective investigations when indicated. Patients with advanced disease are at particularly high risk, and if the clinician is in any doubt, then a CTPA is recommended rather than relying on D-dimer estimation.

Diagnosis for upper extremity thrombosis

The incidence of DVT of the upper extremities is less well established than DVT of the leg but it has been estimated to occur in 2 per 1000 hospital admissions. DVT of the upper extremities can cause morbidity and mortality, similar to DVT of the leg.[50] It is well known that DVT of the upper extremities may be associated with malignant disease and the use of central venous access lines.[51,52]

Diagnostic methods for upper extremity DVT

As for DVT of the leg, contrast venography is generally considered the reference method for diagnosis of DVT of the upper extremities. However, because of its inherent problems, such as availability, use of ionizing radiation, necessity of iodinated contrast media, and technical difficulties in obtaining intravenous access, alternative non-invasive methods have been developed and evaluated.

In contrast to diagnosis of DVT in the legs, few studies have been done in limited numbers of patients to examine the role of ultrasonography in the diagnosis of upper extremity DVT.[52,53] In addition, ultrasonography is potentially problematic because of the anatomy of the upper extremities. The overlying bony structures and inability to visualize more centrally located intrathoracic veins may limit the value of compression ultrasonography. Duplex color ultrasonography has been proposed for diagnosis of DVT of the upper extremities, especially for these areas which are difficult to scan with standard ultrasonography.[54] In a well-designed prospective study, the diagnostic accuracy of duplex color ultrasonography was compared with contrast venography in 126 consecutive in- and outpatients suspected of having DVT of the upper extremities.[55] Contrast venography was obtained after duplex ultrasonography and was judged independently. A three-step protocol, involving compression ultrasonography, color ultrasonography, and color Doppler ultrasonography, was used. Results of ultrasonography were inconclusive in three patients. Venography demonstrated thrombosis in 44 of 99 patients (44 per cent). Importantly, in 36 patients (36 per cent), thrombosis was related to intravenous catheters or malignant disease. Sensitivity and specificity of duplex ultrasonography were 82 per cent (95 per cent CI, 70–93 per cent) and 82 per cent (CI, 72–92 per cent), respectively. Venography and ultrasonography were not feasible in 23 of 126 patients (18 per cent) and 1 of 126 patients (0.8 per cent), respectively. Venous incompressibility correlated well with thrombosis, whereas only 50 per cent of isolated flow abnormalities proved to be thrombosis-related. It was concluded from this study that duplex ultrasonography may be the method of choice for initial diagnosis of patients with suspected thrombosis of the upper extremities. However, in patients with isolated flow abnormalities and in those with a high clinical suspicion, contrast venography should be performed because of the low sensitivity and specificity of abnormal flow.

In a critical review the accuracy of ultrasonography in clinically suspected upper extremity thrombosis,[56] only the above-mentioned study met all of the predefined criteria for adequately evaluating sensitivity and specificity. Overall, the sensitivity of duplex ultrasonography ranged from 56 to 100 per cent, and the specificity ranged from 94 to 100 per cent. No study has evaluated the safety of withholding anticoagulant therapy without additional testing in patients with negative ultrasonography results. The authors conclude that such management studies are needed before a normal ultrasonogram can be used to exclude upper limb DVT and indicate that withholding anticoagulant treatment is safe. In patients with suspected upper extremity DVT, neither a clinical decision rule nor a D-dimer test has been formally evaluated.

Recommended strategies for patients with upper extremity DVT

When a patient presents with upper extremity DVT, color Duplex color ultrasonography is the first test of choice (Fig. 4.7). If this test is normal, a venogram

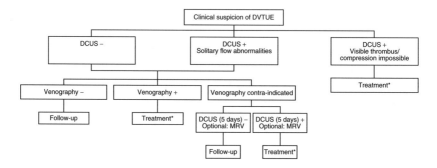

DVTUE = deep vein thrombosis of upper extremity; DCUS = duplex color ultrasonography; * = anticoagulant therapy; MRV = magnetic resonance venography.

Fig. 4.7 Flow diagram for upper extremity DVT diagnosis.[55] Reproduced with kind permission from Springer Science and Business Media. From Baarslag HJ, Koopman MMW, Reekers JA *et al*. Diagnosis and management of deep vein thrombosis of the upper extremities; a systematic review. *European Radiology* 2004;14:1263–74.

should be carried out if there is a high suspicion of DVT. If the ultrasonogram shows solitary flow abnormalities, a venogram is also indicated. If a venogram is contra-indicated, repeat ultrasonography after 5 days is reasonable. The role of CT using contrast or MR venography has not been formally investigated.

Applications for advanced disease

Diagnostic algorithms for diagnosis of VTE are established. However, with the patient having advanced disease, and particularly in those with cancer, there are specific issues to consider. The role of D-dimer estimation is unclear because of its high false positive rate, and the low number of patients with low pre-test clinical probabilities. It seems to play little role in the diagnosis of DVT in cancer patients except to assess which of those with a negative ultrasonogram need to have a repeat scan in a week. Although it has not been formally evaluated in patients with *advanced* cancer as a specific group for the diagnosis of PE, it is likely that CTPA should be the investigation of choice unless pre-test clinical probability is low, as these patients have such a high risk of VTE. A CTPA of chest also may give valuable information in the patient with advanced disease regarding other causes for the patient's breathlessness.

Likewise, although a V/Q test effectively rules out PE, it is less helpful for many patients with cancer or advanced non-malignant disease because of lung or heart disease that would render the scan uninterpretable.

VTE is common and a great symptom mimic in patients with advanced disease. It is a potentially treatable condition that is frequently overlooked. Therefore, a high clinical index of suspicion and a low threshold to investigate appropriately is required.

References

1. Alpert JS, Dalen JE. Epidemiology and natural history of venous thromboembolism. *Progress in Cardiovascular Diseases* 1994;36(6):417–22.
2. Cogo A, Lensing AW, Prandoni P *et al.* Distribution of thrombosis in patients with symptomatic deep vein thrombosis: implications for simplifying the diagnostic process with compression ultrasound. *Archives of Internal Medicine* 1993;153(24):2777–80.
3. Philbrick JT, Becker DM. Calf deep venous thrombosis: a wolf in sheep's clothing? *Archives of Internal Medicine* 1988;148(10):2131–8.
4. Huisman MV, Buller HR, ten Cate JW *et al.* Serial impedance plethysmography for suspected deep venous thrombosis in outpatients: the Amsterdam General Practitioner Study. *The New England Journal of Medicine* 1986;314(13):823–8.
5. Hull RD, Hirsh J, Carter CJ *et al.* Diagnostic efficacy of impedance plethysmography for clinically suspected deep-vein thrombosis: a randomized trial. *Annals of Internal Medicine* 1985;102(1):21–8.
6. Wells PS, Hirsh J, Anderson DR *et al.* Accuracy of clinical assessment of deep-vein thrombosis [published erratum appears in Lancet 1995 Aug 19;346(8973):516] [see comments]. *Lancet* 1995;345(8961):1326–30.

7. Moser KM, LeMoine JR. Is embolic risk conditioned by location of deep venous thrombosis? *Annals of Internal Medicine* 1981;94(4 pt 1):439–44.

8. Huisman MV, Buller HR, ten Cate JW *et al.* Unexpected high prevalence of silent pulmonary embolism in patients with deep venous thrombosis. *Chest* 1989;95(3):498–502.

9. Wells PS. Integrated strategies for the diagnosis of venous thromboembolism. *Journal of Thrombosis and Haemostasis* 2007;5(Suppl 1):41–50.

10. Wells PS, Anderson DR, Rodger M *et al.* Evaluation of D-dimer in the diagnosis of suspected deep-vein thrombosis. *The New England Journal of Medicine* 2003;349(13):1227–35.

11. Tick LW, Ton E, van Voorthuizen T *et al.* Practical diagnostic management of patients with clinically suspected deep vein thrombosis by clinical probability test, compression ultrasonography, and D-dimer test. *The American Journal of Medicine* 2002;113(8):630–5.

12. Wells PS, Anderson DR, Bormanis J *et al.* Value of assessment of pre-test probability of deep-vein thrombosis in clinical management. *Lancet* 1997;350(9094):1795–8.

13. Hull R, Hirsh J, Sackett DL *et al.* Clinical validity of a negative venogram in patients with clinically suspected venous thrombosis. *Circulation* 1981;64(3):622–5.

14. Lensing AW, Prandoni P, Brandjes D *et al.* Detection of deep-vein thrombosis by real-time B-mode ultrasonography [see comments]. *The New England Journal of Medicine* 1989;320(6):342–5.

15. White RH, McGahan JP, Daschbach MM *et al.* Diagnosis of deep-vein thrombosis using duplex ultrasound. *Annals of Internal Medicine* 1989;111(4):297–304.

16. Cronan JJ, Dorfman GS, Scola FH *et al.* Deep venous thrombosis: US assessment using vein compression. *Radiology* 1987;162(1 Pt 1):191–4.

17. Bosson JL, Barro C, Satger B *et al.* Quantitative high D-dimer value is predictive of pulmonary embolism occurrence independently of clinical score in a well-defined low risk factor population. *Journal of Thrombosis and Haemostasis* 2005;3(1):93–9.

18. Righini M, Goehring C, Bounameaux H *et al.* Effects of age on the performance of common diagnostic tests for pulmonary embolism. *The American Journal of Medicine* 2000;109(5):357–61.

19. den Ouden M, Ubachs JM, Stoot JE *et al.* Thrombin-antithrombin III and D-dimer plasma levels in patients with benign or malignant ovarian tumours. *Scandinavian Journal of Clinical and Laboratory Investigation* 1998;58(7):555–9.

20. Gabazza EC, Taguchi O, Yamakami T *et al.* Coagulation-fibrinolysis system and markers of collagen metabolism in lung cancer. *Cancer* 1992;70(11):2631–6.

21. ten Wolde M, Kraaijenhagen RA, Prins MH *et al.* The clinical usefulness of D-dimer testing in cancer patients with suspected deep venous thrombosis. *Archives of Internal Medicine* 2002;162(16):1880–4.

22. Lee AY, Julian JA, Levine MN *et al.* Clinical utility of a rapid whole-blood D-dimer assay in patients with cancer who present with suspected acute deep venous thrombosis. *Annals of Internal Medicine* 1999;131(6):417–23.

23. Di Nisio M, Rutjes AW, Buller HR. Combined use of clinical pre-test probability and D-dimer test in cancer patients with clinically suspected deep venous thrombosis. *Journal of Thrombosis and Haemostasis* 2006;4(1):52–7.

24. Keeling DM, Mackie IJ, Moody A *et al.* The diagnosis of deep vein thrombosis in symptomatic outpatients and the potential for clinical assessment and D-dimer assays to reduce the need for diagnostic imaging. *British Journal of Haematology* 2004;124(1):15–25.

25. Wells PS, Anderson DR, Rodger M *et al.* Derivation of a simple clinical model to categorize patients probability of pulmonary embolism: increasing the models utility with the SimpliRED D-dimer. *Thrombosis and Haemostasis* 2000;83(3):416–20.

26. Wells PS, Anderson DR, Rodger M *et al.* Excluding pulmonary embolism at the bedside without diagnostic imaging: management of patients with suspected pulmonary embolism presenting to the emergency department by using a simple clinical model and d-dimer. *Annals of Internal Medicine* 2001;135(2):98–107.

27. Wicki J, Perneger TV, Junod AF *et al.* Assessing clinical probability of pulmonary embolism in the emergency ward: a simple score. *Archives of Internal Medicine* 2001;161(1):92–7.

28. Le Gal G, Righini M, Roy PM *et al.* Prediction of pulmonary embolism in the emergency department: the revised Geneva score. *Annals of Internal Medicine* 2006;144(3):165–71.

29. Klok FA, Kruisman E, Spaan J *et al.* Comparison of the revised Geneva rule with Wells rule for assessing clinical probability of pulmonary embolism. [Abstract] *Journal of Thrombosis and Haemostasis* 2007;5(Suppl 2),P–M–564.

30. Hudson ER, Smith TP, McDermott VG *et al.* Pulmonary angiography performed with iopamidol: complications in 1,434 patients. *Radiology* 1996;198(1):61–5.

31. Stein PD, Athanasoulis C, Alavi A *et al.* Complications and validity of pulmonary angiography in acute pulmonary embolism. *Circulation* 1992;85(2):462–8.

32. PIOPED. Value of the ventilation/perfusion scan in acute pulmonary embolism. Results of the prospective investigation of pulmonary embolism diagnosis (PIOPED). The PIOPED Investigators [see comments]. *The Journal of the American Medical Association* 1990;263(20):2753–9.

33. Henry JW, Relyea B, Stein PD. Continuing risk of thromboemboli among patients with normal pulmonary angiograms. *Chest* 1995;107(5):1375–8.

34. Hull RD, Hirsh J, Carter CJ *et al.* Pulmonary angiography, ventilation lung scanning, and venography for clinically suspected pulmonary embolism with abnormal perfusion lung scan. *Annals of Internal Medicine* 1983;98(6):891–9.

35. Hayashino Y, Goto M, Noguchi Y *et al.* Ventilation-perfusion scanning and helical CT in suspected pulmonary embolism: meta-analysis of diagnostic performance. *Radiology* 2005;234(3):740–8.

36. Stein PD, Fowler SE, Goodman LR *et al.* Multidetector computed tomography for acute pulmonary embolism. *The New England Journal of Medicine* 2006;354(22):2317–27.

37. van Belle A, Buller HR, Huisman MV *et al.* Effectiveness of managing suspected pulmonary embolism using an algorithm combining clinical probability, D-dimer testing, and computed tomography. *The Journal of the American Medical Association* 2006;295(2):172–9.

38. Anderson DR, Kahn SR, Rodger MA *et al.* Computed tomographic pulmonary angiography vs ventilation-perfusion lung scanning in patients with suspected pulmonary embolism: a randomized controlled trial. *The Journal of the American Medical Association* 2007;298(23):2743–53.

39. Kluge A, Mueller C, Strunk J *et al*. Experience in 207 combined MRI examinations for acute pulmonary embolism and deep vein thrombosis. *AJR American Journal of Roentgenology* 2006;186(6):1686–96.

40. Peak AS, Sheller A. Risk factors for developing gadolinium-induced nephrogenic systemic fibrosis. *The Annals of Pharmacotherapy* 2007;41(9):1481–5.

41. Oudkerk M, van Beek EJ, Wieloploski P *et al*. Comparison of contrast-enhanced magnetic resonance angiography and conventional pulmonary angiography for the diagnosis of pulmonary embolism: a prospective study. *Lancet* 2002;(359):1643–7.

42. Anderson DR, Kovacs MJ, Kovacs G *et al*. Combined use of clinical assessment and D-dimer to improve the management of patients presenting to the emergency department with suspected deep vein thrombosis (the EDITED Study). *Journal of Thrombosis and Haemostasis* 2003;1(4):645–51.

43. Bernardi E, Prandoni P, Lensing AW *et al*. D-dimer testing as an adjunct to ultrasonography in patients with clinically suspected deep vein thrombosis: prospective cohort study. The Multicentre Italian D-dimer Ultrasound Study Investigators Group. *British Medical Journal* 1998;317(7165):1037–40.

44. Kraaijenhagen RA, Piovella F, Bernardi E *et al*. Simplification of the diagnostic management of suspected deep vein thrombosis. *Archives of Internal Medicine* 2002;162(8):907–11.

45. Ghanima W, Almaas V, Aballi S *et al*. Management of suspected pulmonary embolism (PE) by D-dimer and multi-slice computed tomography in outpatients: an outcome study. *Journal of Thrombosis and Haemostasis* 2005;3(9):1926–32.

46. Goekoop RJ, Steeghs N, Niessen RW *et al*. Simple and safe exclusion of pulmonary embolism in outpatients using quantitative D-dimer and Wells' simplified decision rule. *Thrombosis and Haemostasis* 2007;97(1):146–50.

47. Di Nisio M, Sohne M, Kamphuisen PW *et al*. D-Dimer test in cancer patients with suspected acute pulmonary embolism. *Journal of Thrombosis and Haemostasis* 2005;3(6):1239–42.

48. Righini M, Le Gal G, De Lucia S *et al*. Clinical usefulness of D-dimer testing in cancer patients with suspected pulmonary embolism. *Thrombosis and Haemostasis* 2006;95(4):715–9.

49. Sohne M, Kruip MJ, Nijkeuter M *et al*. Accuracy of clinical decision rule, D-dimer and spiral computed tomography in patients with malignancy, previous venous thromboembolism, COPD or heart failure and in older patients with suspected pulmonary embolism. *Journal of Thrombosis and Haemostasis* 2006;4(5):1042–6.

50. Prandoni P, Polistena P, Bernardi E *et al*. Upper-extremity deep vein thrombosis. Risk factors, diagnosis, and complications [see comments]. *Archives of Internal Medicine* 1997;157(1):57–62.

51. Girolami A, Prandoni P, Zanon E *et al*. Venous thromboses of upper limbs are more frequently associated with occult cancer as compared with those of lower limbs. *Blood Coagulation and Fibrinolysis* 1999;10(8):455–7.

52. Falk RL, Smith DF. Thrombosis of upper extremity thoracic inlet veins: diagnosis with duplex Doppler sonography. *AJR American Journal of Roentgenology* 1987;149(4):677–82.

53. Knudson GJ, Wiedmeyer DA, Erickson SJ *et al.* Color Doppler sonographic imaging in the assessment of upper-extremity deep venous thrombosis. *AJR American Journal of Roentgenology* 1990;154(2):399–403.

54. Haire WD, Lynch TG, Lieberman RP *et al.* Utility of duplex ultrasound in the diagnosis of asymptomatic catheter- induced subclavian vein thrombosis. *Journal of Ultrasound in Medicine* 1991;10(9):493–6.

55. Baarslag, HJ, Koopman, MMW, Reekers, JA *et al.* Diagnosis and management of deep venous thrombosis of the upper extremities: a review. *European Radiology* 2004; (14), 1263–74.

56. Mustafa BO, Rathbun SW, Whitsett TL *et al.* Sensitivity and specificity of ultraso nography in the diagnosis of upper extremity deep vein thrombosis: a systematic review. *Archives of Internal Medicine* 2002;162(4):401–4.

Chapter 5

Anticoagulants: current and future therapeutic options

Robert Weinkove and Beverley J. Hunt

Introduction

For 50 years, the options for therapeutic anticoagulation were limited to unfractionated heparin and oral vitamin K antagonists (coumarins). Although they are highly effective anticoagulants, both drugs have drawbacks. Unfractionated heparin is only active parenterally, has a short half-life and has the capacity to cause a life-threatening complication; heparin-induced thrombocytopenia (HIT). Coumarins have multiple food and drug interactions and a slow onset of action. Both classes of drug have narrow therapeutic ranges, substantial inter-individual dose variability, and require routine therapeutic drug monitoring.

The emergence of low molecular weight heparins (LMWH) in the 1980s represented a substantial advancement in therapeutic anticoagulation. Compared to unfractionated heparin, they offer more predictable pharmacokinetics, less frequent dosage, a lower frequency of HIT, and no requirement for routine therapeutic monitoring. LMWH appear to be safe in long-term use, and are of particular value in the setting of cancer, where studies have indicated lower bleeding and thrombosis risks than with the oral vitamin K antagonists.

The 1990s saw the emergence of a number of new parenteral anticoagulants (some of which are unavailable in the UK) including the synthetic heparin derivatives fondaparinux and idraparinux, and the direct thrombin inhibitors argatroban, hirudin, and bivalirudin. Fondaparinux appears to have similar efficacy to LMWH and has no capacity to cause HIT. Idraparinux has the additional benefit of a very long half-life permitting once-weekly administration. Hirudin has proved useful in the management of HIT, but widespread use has been limited by the requirement for therapeutic drug monitoring and the high dependence of clearance upon renal function. Bivalirudin and argatroban have very short half-lives, and their use has been largely restricted to percutaneous coronary procedures and the management of HIT.

The next decade will see the emergence of a new generation of oral antico-agulants that do not require routine therapeutic monitoring. This will facilitate long-term outpatient thromboprophylaxis and may lead to substantial changes in the thresholds for starting therapeutic and prophylactic anticoagulation, and in the recommended duration of anticoagulation.

The new oral anticoagulants present their own challenges: long-term effects and unexpected drug interactions may emerge, there are no specific reversal agents in case of bleeding, and the cost of the newer agents may eliminate any savings made by omitting therapeutic drug monitoring. Once the need for routine therapeutic drug monitoring is eliminated, the responsibility for initiation and review of anticoagulation may increasingly move from secondary care to primary care providers. This will bring substantial changes to the shape of anticoagulant services.

This chapter aims to review the pharmacology and use of both the established and the newer anticoagulants, to discuss specific issues in the field of palliative care, and to present illustrative case studies.

General overview of the subject

Unfractionated heparin

History

Heparin was one of a number of anticoagulants first isolated between 1916 and 1922 by medical students Jay McLean and Emmett Holt in William Howell's laboratory at Johns Hopkins University. As the source of the preparation was canine liver, Howell named it heparin after the Greek word for liver, 'ηπαρ' or 'hepar'.[1]

In the 1930s, researchers at the Connaught Medical Research Laboratories in Toronto and at the Karolinska Institute in Stockholm purified heparin and used it as an anticoagulant in human trials. The clinical use of heparin became widespread after the Second World War.

Composition

Unfractionated heparin (UFH) is a naturally occurring glycosaminoglycan produced by mast cells and basophils. The pharmaceutical product is derived from tissues rich in mast cells such as porcine intestine or bovine lung.

The heparin molecule is a polymer of repeating disaccharide units, primarily comprising sulphated glucosamine and uronic acid. Heparin is a heterogeneous mixture of differing chain lengths, but most current preparations have a mean molecular weight of 13,000–15,000 Da.[2]

Mechanism of action and pharmacology

The anticoagulant activity of heparin is mediated by endogenous antithrombin, a physiological inhibitor of coagulation. A specific pentasaccharide sequence of the heparin molecule binds to antithrombin, inducing a conformational change and a 1000-fold increase in antithrombin activity. In turn, antithrombin inhibits thrombin and factor Xa, both essential factors for normal coagulation. Only the pentasaccharide sequence is required for the inhibition of factor Xa (anti-Xa activity), whereas a longer sequence of 18 saccharides, including the pentasaccharide, is necessary for thrombin inhibition.

Pharmacological heparins differ in their anticoagulant activity depending on the distribution of heparin chain molecular weights. The activity of heparins is standardized in either International Units (IU) as determined by the World Health Organization international standard, or United States Pharmacopeial (USP) units.

Heparins are only active when administered parenterally. UFH can be given intravenously or subcutaneously; intramuscular administration should be avoided as it can result in large haematomas. At typical therapeutic doses, the half-life of intravenous UFH is 45–60 minutes, demanding continuous intravenous infusion for effective anticoagulation. UFH, given subcutaneously, has a lower bioavailability than intravenous heparin. By the subcutaneous route, UFH activity starts at 2 hours and lasts for approximately 10 hours, necessitating twice-daily dosage.[3]

Dosage

Treatment of VTE with intravenous UFH is usually initiated with an intravenous bolus over 5 minutes (75 IU/kg, or 5000 IU for a 70 kg adult) followed by continuous intravenous infusion (18 IU/kg/h). The activated partial thromboplastin time ratio (APTT-R) is measured 4–6 hours after commencing the infusion, and the rate of infusion adjusted accordingly.

Treatment doses of UFH can also be administered subcutaneously for the treatment of deep vein thrombosis,[4] in which case an intravenous bolus should be given initially (dosage as above), followed immediately by the first of subsequent 12-hourly subcutaneous injections of UFH 250 IU/kg. If therapeutic monitoring is used, the APTT ratio should be checked 4–6 hours after subcutaneous injection and the next dose adjusted accordingly. The therapeutic range is the same as for intravenous heparin.

Subcutaneous UFH has also been used for the treatment of acute venous thrombosis without APTT monitoring. Patients given an initial dose of 333 IU/kg UFH followed by a fixed dose of 250 IU/kg 12-hourly without

APTT-guided dose adjustment had similar clinical outcomes and bleeding rates to those treated with LMWH.[5]

Prophylactic doses of subcutaneous UFH range from 5000 to 7500 IU bd. APTT monitoring is not required when prophylactic doses are used, but the platelet count should be monitored as HIT can occur.

Monitoring

As there is a narrow therapeutic range and wide variability in response to a given dose of heparin, treatment doses typically require frequent monitoring and dose adjustment.

Heparin is usually monitored using the APTT, which is sensitive to both thrombin and factor Xa inhibition. The APTT can be expressed in seconds or as a ratio to a control APTT. An APTT-R of 1.5–2.5 is usually associated with therapeutic anticoagulation, but because APTT reagents have differing heparin sensitivity, local reference ranges should be used.[6]

In patients receiving UFH, the APTT-R should be monitored and the infusion rate adjusted until a therapeutic value is obtained. Thereafter, the APTT-R should be monitored at least once every 24 hours, as heparin requirements can change rapidly over time. Heparin dose adjustment protocols that reflect local target APTT ranges should be used.[7]

The platelet count should be checked before starting UFH and repeated at least every other day between days 4 and 14 of UFH treatment. If the patient has received heparin within the last 100 days, platelet count monitoring should begin earlier, within 24 hours of starting heparin.[8] This is to monitor HIT (see section 'Adverse effects' below).

Reversal

As intravenous UFH has a short half-life, cessation of the infusion is usually sufficient for the management of mild bleeding symptoms. For more severe bleeding, rapid reversal of the anticoagulant activity of UFH can be achieved with protamine sulphate. 1 mg protamine is administered for every 100 IU of heparin given within the previous hour up to a maximum of 40–50 mg protamine. The dose can be repeated if necessary. Protamine is a protein derived from fish milt, and can lead to allergic reactions. Pre-treatment with corticosteroids and antihistamines may be warranted in patients with a known fish allergy.

Indications and contraindications

For the treatment of venous thromboembolism (VTE), UFH has been largely superseded by LMWH that offer more reliable pharmacokinetics and more convenient dosage. However, UFH may be of particular use in patients with renal failure (where LMWH clearance is reduced) or perhaps in palliative care patients who require emergency surgery and require short-term anticoagulation that can be quickly reversed. Treatment doses of UFH are indicated for the treatment of venous and arterial thrombosis, for acute coronary syndromes, and postoperatively after vascular reconstructive surgery. Prophylactic subcutaneous doses of UFH are also indicated for the prophylaxis of VTE. However, their role in the palliative setting is limited.

The only absolute contraindications to heparin are current major bleeding or confirmed history of HIT (especially if in the last 100 days). Relative contraindications include an unconfirmed prior history of HIT or potential bleeding risk such as: uncontrolled severe hypertension, active peptic ulcer, recent trauma or surgery to the brain, orbit or spinal cord, recent stroke, recent intracranial haemorrhage, thrombocytopenia, or other bleeding diathesis. Treatment doses of heparin should be avoided in patients undergoing epidural or spinal anaesthesia.

Adverse effects

A slight fall in platelet count (of <30 per cent compared to baseline) occurs in up to one-third of patients within the first 4 days of starting heparin. This is a reversible dose-dependent phenomenon, is not associated with bleeding or thrombotic complications, and does not require cessation of heparin.

More marked falls in platelet count (of >50 per cent compared to baseline) should raise the possibility of HIT. HIT is a life-threatening complication of heparin treatment and occurs in 0.3–6.5 per cent of those receiving UFH. The onset is typically between 5 and 10 days after starting UFH unless heparin has previously been administered, in which case it may begin earlier. The cause is development of an IgG antibody to heparin and platelet factor 4, which forms a complex capable of activating and depleting platelets. Because the thrombocytopenia is due to platelet activation, patients with HIT are paradoxically at high risk of both venous and arterial thrombosis; bleeding is rare. Other features may include necrotizing skin changes at heparin injection sites or a history of anaphylactoid reactions to heparin injection. A clinical scoring system for suspected HIT has been developed and can be useful in determining the need for further investigation.[9]

The diagnosis of HIT may be confirmed by specific enzyme-linked immunosorbant assay (ELISA) or by functional platelet studies. The treatment is immediate cessation of all heparins (including line flushes and including LMWH) and initiation of an alternative anticoagulant such as danaparoid, hirudin, or fondaparinux at therapeutic doses. Platelet transfusion is contraindicated, and warfarin should not be started until the platelet count has recovered, as it may cause microvascular necrosis.[8]

Prolonged use of heparin can lead to osteopenia or osteoporosis by increasing osteoclast activity and reducing osteoblast numbers. Two to three per cent of patients receiving treatment dose UFH for more than 1 month developed vertebral fractures. The risk of osteoporosis is lower for low molecular weight than for UFH.[10]

As with all anticoagulants, heparin can lead to bleeding. The monitoring and reversal of UFH are discussed above. Injection site and hypersensitivity reactions are described with all heparins, and may necessitate a use of an alternative anticoagulant.

LMWH

History

LMWH are produced by the enzymatic or chemical depolymerization of UFH. Since their introduction in the 1980s, LMWH have largely superseded UFH by virtue of their more predictable pharmacokinetic profiles, less frequent dosage, and a lower incidence of adverse effects.

Composition

LMWH are produced by enzymatic or chemical fractionation of crude heparin. The commercially available products possess mean molecular weights in the range of 3,000–5,000 Da. The molecular weights, anti-Xa/anti-IIa ratios and half-lives of some commercially available LMWH preparations are given in Table 5.1.

Mechanism of action and pharmacology

Like UFH, the anticoagulant activity of LMWH is mediated by antithrombin. Whilst antithrombin-bound UFH can inhibit both activated thrombin (factor IIa)

Table 5.1 Molecular weights, anti-Xa/IIa ratio, and half-lives of some LMWH preparations.

LMWH	Mean molecular weight (Da)	Anti-Xa/anti-IIa ratio	t$_{1/2}$ after subcutaneous administration (hours)
Bemiparin	2,900	9.6	5–6
Enoxaparin	3,200	3.9	4–5
Nadroparin	3,600	3.3	3–4
Tinzaparin	4,800	1.6	3–4
Dalteparin	5,000	2.5	3–5
UFH	14,000	1.0	—

and factor Xa, LMWH have anti-Xa activity but offer little or no thrombin inhibition. An antithrombin-binding pentasaccharide sequence alone is required for the inhibition of factor Xa (anti-Xa activity), whereas a longer sequence of 18 saccharides, including the pentasaccharide, is required for the bridging function necessary to inhibit thrombin. This explains the higher ratio of anti-Xa to anti-IIa activity of smaller LMWH molecules.

In contrast with UFH, which is rapidly cleared by the reticuloendothelial system, LMWH are cleared slowly by a renal mechanism. In individuals with normal renal function, the bioavailability and clearance of subcutaneous LMWH are sufficiently predictable to allow dosage without monitoring.

LMWH are administered subcutaneously. Various products have differing pharmacokinetics and relative anti-Xa / anti-IIa activities depending upon their molecular weight.

Dosage

LMWH should be dosed according to the manufacturer's instructions. Treatment doses of LMWH are dosed according to body weight, whilst prophylactic doses are usually fixed. Although LMWH have low lipid solubility and are highly plasma protein-bound, the pharmacokinetics of LMWH are remarkably predictable in obese patients. Pharmacokinetic studies indicate that LMWH can be dosed by total body weight and need not be capped in obese patients.[11] Anti-Xa monitoring can be used in patients with very high body weight. An alternative strategy is to dose according to total body weight and to reduce the dose if bleeding occurs.

The fixed doses of LMWH used for thromboprophylaxis may be insufficient for obese patients, for whom an empiric dose increase or a weight-adjusted thromboprophylactic dose may be appropriate.[12]

Given the renal clearance of LMWH, it is not surprising that both peak anti-Xa activity and half-life are increased in patients with renal failure. Even when prophylactic doses are used, anti-Xa activity accumulates after prolonged use of LMWH. Bleeding complications are more common in LMWH-treated patients with renal failure.[13] In those with severe renal failure (creatinine clearance <30 mL/min), dose adjustment is necessary and should be guided by monitoring of the anti-Xa level. Alternatively, another anticoagulant such as UFH could be used.

Monitoring

One of the advantages of LMWH is that routine monitoring is not necessary. However, LMWH monitoring is often indicated in patients with progressive cancer since body weight, renal clearance, serum albumin, and thrombogenicity are likely to change over time. The patient with progressive cancer may need to have the weight-adjusted dose recalculated in the light of weight loss. LMWH monitoring should also be considered for patients with deteriorating renal functional though the majority of patients with such progressive disease are likely to be receiving symptomatic support only. There may be some patients with comorbid chronic renal failure and otherwise reasonable performance status, for whom therapeutic anticoagulation is considered appropriate, and in these patients, LMWH should be monitored or alternative anticoagulants should be considered.

The APTT is not sufficiently sensitive to anti-Xa activity to permit monitoring. Therapeutic monitoring of LMWH therefore requires the direct measurement of plasma anti-Xa activity. Because of the risk of HIT, patients receiving LMWH should have a baseline platelet count on the day of starting treatment, and platelet counts every 2–4 days between days 4 and 14 of treatment.[8]

Reversal

Most bleeding complications are mild and can be managed by dose reduction or cessation of LMWH. For severe bleeding, partial reversal of the anticoagulant activity of LMWH can be achieved with protamine sulphate. Administration of 1 mg protamine for every 100 IU of LMWH given within the previous 8 hours (maximum 40–50 mg protamine) can reverse up to 90 per cent of anti-IIa and 60 per cent of anti-Xa activity.

A partial return of LMWH anticoagulant activity may be seen 3 hours after reversal due to continued LMWH absorption from the subcutaneous injection site. Protamine can be re-administered if necessary.

Indications and contraindications

LMWH are licensed for the treatment of VTE, for prophylaxis of VTE, and for the management of acute coronary syndromes.

Absolute contraindications to LMWH include active major haemorrhage or recent HIT. Relative contraindications include increased bleeding risk, hypersensitivity to other heparins, and renal impairment (creatinine clearance <30 mL/Min). Caution is required when using LMWH in patients undergoing invasive procedures, especially epidural or intrathecal anaesthesia, as bleeding risk is increased. If a patient receiving therapeutic doses of LMWH requires an invasive procedure with a significant risk of haemorrhage, the interval between the last LMWH dose and the intervention should be maximized, and should be at least 12 hours unless clinical urgency dictates otherwise.

Adverse effects

HIT is a known adverse effect of LMWH. The rate of HIT may be lower for LMWH than for UFH when thromboprophylactic doses are used[14] but appears to be similar to UFH at treatment doses.[15]

The risk of osteoporosis with prolonged use of LMWH is substantially lower than with UFH. The reason for this may be that unlike UFH, LMWH do not stimulate osteoclast activity, although both LMWH and UFH have adverse effects on osteoblast numbers.[16] There is little data on osteoporosis within the palliative population. One small cohort of advanced cancer patients receiving long-term treatment dose of LMWH reported no clinical evidence of osteoporosis although the numbers (62 patients) were too small to draw any firm conclusions.[17] As with all anticoagulants, LMWH can lead to bleeding. LMWH reversal is discussed above.

Patients with cutaneous reactions to LMWH may tolerate other LMWH formulations or danaparoid, but cross-reactivity rates are high. Fondaparinux is a useful alternative in this scenario.[18]

Danaparoid

Danaparoid sodium is a low molecular weight heparinoid derived from animal intestinal mucosa. It is a mixture of heparin, dermatan, and chondroitin sulphates, and like LMWH inhibits factor Xa via antithrombin. Danaparoid is administered parenterally, either intravenously or subcutaneously, and has an elimination half-life of 24 hours. Danaparoid has the advantage of a low cross-reactivity rate with HIT antibodies, and is used primarily for the treatment of HIT.

Danaparoid has very little anti-IIa activity, with a Xa/IIa ratio approximately 28. Therapeutic monitoring therefore requires measurement of the anti-Xa level, with a typical target range of 0.5–0.8 U/mL for the treatment of VTE.[19] There is no specific reversal agent for danaparoid—it is not neutralized by protamine sulphate.

To date, its use in the palliative setting has been limited to patients with HIT although emerging data within the cancer population may lead to increased usage.

Coumarins

History

Anticoagulant coumarins were first isolated by Karl Paul Link at the University of Wisconsin in the 1930s. The observation that cows bled to death after eating mouldy sweet clover had lead Link's team to isolate the anticoagulant factor from the contaminated clover. Link later developed a synthetic coumarin derivative. This was patented by the Wisconsin Alumni Research Foundation who named it warfarin as a contraction of the organization's acronym, WARF, and the word coumarin. The therapeutic use of coumarins in humans became widespread in the 1940s.[20]

A number of other coumarins have been used as oral anticoagulants, including dicoumarol, acenocoumarol, phenprocoumon, and phenindione. All have similar mechanisms of action and adverse effects to warfarin, but the drugs differ in dosage, half-life, and to some extent in their drug interactions.

Mechanism of action and pharmacology

The coagulation factors II, VII, IX, and X, as well as the naturally occurring anticoagulants protein C and S are dependent upon vitamin K. In each case, synthesis of the functional protein requires the post-translational γ-carboxylation of N-terminal glutamine residues.

During the γ-carboxylation step, reduced vitamin K is oxidized to vitamin K epoxide. Vitamin K epoxide is recycled to reduced vitamin K via a two-step pathway requiring the enzymes vitamin K epoxide reductase and vitamin K reductase. Vitamin K epoxide reductase is inhibited by coumarin anticoagulants. Coumarins therefore result in the production of inactive noncarboxylated forms of factors II, VII, IX, and X as well as factors C and S.

Warfarin has an oral bioavailability approaching 100 per cent. Peak serum concentrations are reached around three hours of oral administration and the half-life is 36–42 hours. Warfarin is highly protein-bound, mainly to albumin. Despite rapid absorption of warfarin and other coumarins, the onset of the anticoagulant effect is delayed as it requires the gradual depletion of functional coagulation factors. Metabolism is hepatic, requiring the cytochrome P450 2C9 hepatic microsomal enzyme.

Interactions

For patients with advanced disease drug, interactions can be a major problem since the changing symptomatology of progressive disease will necessitate frequent medication changes and the ongoing challenges of managing polypharmacy. Likewise, changing appetite and nutritional intake (including food supplements) may alter the ingestion of foods rich in vitamin K1 (phytomenadione), which will reduce the efficacy of coumarins by overcoming its inhibition of vitamin K recycling. Examples of vitamin K1-rich foods include green leafy vegetables such as cabbage, chard, and spinach, cauliflower, broccoli, liver, chick peas, and olive oil.

Numerous drugs and herbal remedies are known to interact with coumarins and alter the anticoagulant effect. Although concomitant use of interacting drugs with coumarins is not contraindicated, close therapeutic monitoring is required when these medications are started or stopped, or when doses are changed. A nonexhaustive list of interactions with warfarin is given in Table 5.2.

In addition to the interactions above, the concomitant use of other anticoagulants and antiplatelet agents, including nonsteroidal anti-inflammatory drugs, can lead to an increase in bleeding risk in patients taking warfarin.

Dosage

The anticoagulant activity of coumarins is not established immediately, as depletion of the normal coagulation factors takes several days. For patients requiring rapid anticoagulation, an alternative anticoagulant (such as LMWH) should be used during coumarin loading.

Schedules for coumarin initiation can be divided into high-dose loading schedules, which are useful for patients requiring rapid anticoagulation such as those with active thrombosis, and low-dose loading schedules, which are useful for patients without active thrombosis such as those with uncomplicated atrial fibrillation.

Initiation of coumarins with high-dose loading schedules regimen for warfarin requires daily international normalized ratio (INR) monitoring. Such loading schedules can create a temporary pro-thrombotic state. This is because as far as depleting the coagulation factors II, VII, IX, and X, coumarins also deplete protein C and S, naturally occuring inhibitors of coagulation. The half-life of protein C is short, and as a consequence during the first few days of coumarin therapy, patients may be rendered protein C deficient before coagulation factor levels fall sufficiently to prevent thrombosis. This temporary

Table 5.2 Common drug interactions with warfarin (see BNF for full list of interactions).

Potentiation of warfarin	Inhibition of warfarin
Antifungals: fluconazole, itraconazole, ketoconazole	Antiepileptics: carbamazepine, phenytoin Antifungal: griseofulvin
Antibiotics: chloramphenicol, ciprofloxacin, clarithromycin erythromycin, metronidazole, norfloxacin, tetracyclines, ofloxacin, sulphonamides	Antituberculous agents: rifampicin
Antituberculous agents: isoniazid	Others: barbiturates, colestyramine, chronic alcohol use, vitamin K
Antidysrhythmics: amiodarone, propafenone	
Others: tamoxifen, fluorouracil, omeprazole, cimetidine, acute alcohol use, sulphinpyrazone, thyroid hormones	

pro-thrombotic state can be avoided by continuing LMWH or a similar anti-coagulant until the INR has been in the therapeutic range for at least 2 days.

Some individuals are highly sensitive to coumarins. A 50 per cent reduction of loading dose should be considered in malnourished patients, in the elderly, in those with liver disease or a pre-existing coagulopathy, or patients taking medications that potentiate coumarin activity. Clinicians should refer to local guidelines for current practice.

Some invasive procedures such as dental extractions and bone marrow biopsies can be safely performed without stopping coumarin anticoagulation provided the INR is in the therapeutic range. For most surgery, however, coumarins should be stopped 4 days beforehand to allow sufficient time for normalization of the INR. If the patient requires continued anticoagulation, an alternative such as a LMWH can be used during the perioperative period.

Monitoring

Because of the considerable inter-individual variability in dose requirements, and the myriad food and drug interactions, coumarins require routine thera-peutic monitoring. Patients with advanced cancer are likely to require intensive monitoring, which may have a detrimental effect on their quality of life.[21] The pro-thrombin time (PT) is the principal coagulation test used to monitor coumarins, as it reflects the levels of three of the four clotting factors affected by coumarins (factors II, VII, and IX). The PT is measured in seconds, and can be reported as a ratio to that of a control sample (PT ratio).

To provide inter-laboratory consistency in coumarin monitoring and target ranges, a calibration model based on a WHO standard is used to convert the locally measured PT ratio into an INR.

Near-patient testing devices for INR monitoring are now available, allowing patients to monitor their own INR at home and even to determine their own coumarin dose adjustments. It is recommended that self-monitoring of coumarins takes place within a structured programme involving patient education, quality assurance, and clinical support.[22]

Reversal

Administration of vitamin K_1 can reverse the anticoagulant effects of coumarins. The reversal of coumarins with vitamin K1 takes at least 6 hours, as it necessitates the *de novo* production of active γ-carboxylated coagulation factors by the liver. In patients with advanced disease, this may take even longer.

A dose of 10 mg vitamin K, either orally or intravenously, is usually sufficient for coumarin reversal. This dose will, however, make anticoagulation with coumarins difficult during the following 2 weeks. Lower doses of 2–5 mg vitamin K may therefore be preferable in patients without life-threatening bleeding.

Intramuscular administration of vitamin K should be avoided due to the risk of haematoma formation.

Immediate reversal of warfarin can be achieved with direct replacement of the coagulation factors. Fresh frozen plasma (FFP) contains all the vitamin K-dependent coagulation factors, and can reverse warfarin when given at a dose of 15–20 ml/kg. As the half-life of certain factors (especially factor VII) is short, vitamin K replacement should be given concomitantly.

Pro-thrombin complex concentrates (PCC) are plasma-derived products containing the vitamin K-dependent coagulation factors in a concentrated form. The activity of PCC is usually expressed in terms of units of factor IX, the typical dose required for warfarin reversal being 20 IU/kg. PCC are given as a slow intravenous push over several minutes. Although more expensive than FFP, PCC have the advantage of a small volume of administration, rapid preparation (no thawing required), rapid administration, and more complete reversal of warfarin activity. As with FFP, vitamin K replacement should be given in conjunction with PCC.

Indications and contraindications

Common clinical indications for coumarins include prevention of arterial thrombosis in patients with atrial fibrillation, mechanical heart valves or severe peripheral arterial disease, and prevention and treatment of recurrent venous thrombosis.

The target INR range varies according to clinical indication (see Table 5.3).

Coumarins are relatively contraindicated in patients at increased risk of bleeding, for example, in those with uncontrolled severe hypertension, active peptic ulcer, recent trauma or surgery to the brain, orbit, or spinal cord, recent

Table 5.3 Typical target INR ranges for anticoagulation with coumarins.

Indication	Typical target INR
Atrial fibrillation	2.5
Venous thrombosis	2.5
Recurrent venous thrombosis whilst off anticoagulation	2.5
Recurrent venous thrombosis whilst on therapeutic anticoagulation	3.5
Antiphospholipid syndrome with arterial thrombosis	3.0–4.0
Mechanical heart valve	2.0–4.5 (depending upon valve type and location)

ischaemic stroke (within last 14 days), recent intracranial haemorrhage, thrombocytopenia, or other bleeding diathesis. In the advanced cancer population, coumarins are associated with a high incidence of bleeding complications even with frequent monitoring.[23]

Adverse effects

The principal adverse effect of coumarins is bleeding, with a risk of fatal haemorrhage of 0.25 per cent per year in unselected patients.[24] This risk appears higher in patients with cancer,[25] in whom multiple interacting medications, hypoalbuminaemia, weight loss, and other haemorrhagic diatheses may contribute to a higher bleeding rate. There is also evidence to suggest that the bleeding tendency increases with disease progression even at therapeutic INR.[26]

While there remains an established role for coumarins in the anticoagulation of patients with advanced non-malignant disease, its role on advanced cancer patients has largely been superseded by LMWH. LMWH have several benefits over warfarin in this setting, including reduced re-thrombosis risk,[27] lack of requirement for therapeutic drug monitoring, less variability in efficacy due to changes in nutritional status, and fewer drug interactions.

Although most patients with advanced cancer find LMWH an acceptable long-term treatment, some will find the daily injection burdensome.[21] Although warfarin is less efficacious than LMWH, it may be the preferred option for some patients having balanced the potential hazards of coumarin use with a desire to avoid daily injections.

Synthetic pentasaccharides

Fondaparinux

Fondaparinux is a synthetic drug consisting of the antithrombin-binding pentasaccharide sequence found in the heparin molecule. Like LMWH, fondaparinux binds the antithrombin molecule causing a conformational change, which enhances its activity against factor Xa. Because there are no additional saccharides to provide the necessary bridging function for thrombin binding, fondaparinux has no activity against thrombin.

Fondaparinux is given as a subcutaneous injection and has a half-life of 17 hours, making it suitable for once-daily dosage. Clearance is exclusively renal, so dose adjustment in renal failure is required and it is not recommended in those with a creatinine clearance of <30 mL/min. Fondaparinux does not bind to platelet factor IV, so has no capacity to cause HIT. Fondaparinux is licensed for the treatment of HIT and can be safely given to patients with a prior history of HIT.

The dosage is 2.5 mg subcutaneously once daily for VTE prophylaxis or 7.5 mg subcutaneously (50–100kg person) once daily for treatment of VTE or acute coronary syndromes.

Routine monitoring of fondaparinux is not necessary, but in specific situations such as renal impairment or in those with extremes of body mass index, the anticoagulant activity can be monitored using anti-Xa levels (see section 'LMWH' above).

There is no specific reversal agent for fondaparinux—protamine sulphate is ineffective. In the setting of fondaparinux-associated bleeding, blood product support can be given. Experimental data indicate that recombinant activated factor VII may partially reverse the anticoagulant effect of fondaparinux.[28]

Idraparinux

Idraparinux is a methylated sulphated derivative of fondaparinux with very high affinity for antithrombin. This results in a half-life of 80–130 hours, similar to that of the antithrombin molecule itself, and enables once-weekly subcutaneous dosage. The dose used in current phase III trials for treatment of VTE is 2.5 mg subcutaneously once weekly. However, the Van Gogh studies have shown there was a higher rate of recurrence in those treated for pulmonary embolism and an excess of deaths at 6 months (6.4 per cent versus 4.4 per cent P=0.04) compared to standard treatment.[29] When the same investigators compared the use of idraparinux versus placebo for 6 months in extended thromboprophylaxis in over 1,000 patients after 6 months standard treatment for VTE, they found a major bleeding rate of 3.1 per cent versus 0.9 per cent.[30] A trial of idraparinux 2.5 mg weekly versus warfarin in patients with atrial fibrillation was terminated because there was excessive bleeding when compared to warfarin. Based on this evidence, there is likely to be a limited role for this drug within the palliative care setting.

Recently, a biotinylated form of idraparinux has been introduced into clinical trials. The addition of biotin to idraparinux enables neutralization of the anticoagulant effect by the administration of avidin, providing a potentially useful approach to reverse the effects of idraparinux in patients with serious bleeding.

Parenteral direct thrombin inhibitors

Unlike heparins, direct thrombin inhibitors are not dependent on endogenous antithrombin for their anticoagulant effects.

Hirudin

Hirudin is a 65-amino acid polypeptide, originally discovered in the saliva of the medicinal leech, *Hirudo medicinalis*. Two recombinant derivatives are available: lepirudin and desirudin. Hirudin is an irreversible direct thrombin inhibitor, binding to both the active and substrate recognition sites of the thrombin molecule. Hirudins are usually given as intravenous infusions. It is not active orally.

As the clearance of hirudin is exclusively renal, the half-life is highly dependent on renal function. With normal renal function, hirudin has a half-life of 60 minutes after intravenous administration, but in those with end-stage renal failure, the half-life can be as long as 300 hours.

Hirudin requires therapeutic monitoring. The APTT is usually used, with a typical target APTT ratio of 2.0–2.5. The ecarin clotting time may be better alternative for hirudin monitoring, but is less widely available.

Hirudin is licensed for the treatment of thrombosis associated with HIT. Its major adverse effect is bleeding. Within a week's treatment, 40–70 per cent of patients develop hirudin antibodies. The antibodies are sometimes inhibitory, but may bind to hirudin and reduce renal clearance, resulting in a prolongation of half-life and an increase in the anticoagulant effect.[31]

There is no specific reversal agent for hirudin. Options in bleeding patients include blood product support, activated pro-thrombin complex concentrates (APCC) or recombinant activated factor VII. Hirudin is not cleared by haemodialysis and its indication in the advanced disease setting, beyond the management of complications such as HIT are yet to be established.

Bivalirudin

Bivalirudin is a recombinant 20-amino acid polypeptide analogue of hirudin. It binds to the substrate binding site of thrombin, but unlike hirudin, can be cleaved by thrombin itself, making bivalirudin a reversible thrombin inhibitor. Bivalirudin has a half-life of 25 minutes following intravenous injection. Because only a proportion of excretion is renal, clearance is less-dependent upon renal function than for hirudin. Bivalirudin is monitored using the APTT or ecarin clotting time.

Because of its short half-life, the clinical use of bivalirudin is usually restricted to the management of acute coronary symptoms and to anticoagulation during percutaneous coronary intervention.

There is no specific reversal agent for bivalirudin. Because of the short half-life, bleeding can be managed with blood product support alone until the anticoagulant activity declines.

Argatroban

Argatroban is a small molecule reversible thrombin inhibitor derived from the amino acid arginine. It is only active parenterally. The half-life is around

40 minutes, and clearance is primarily hepatic. Dose adjustment is recommended in those with moderate liver failure. Argatroban is monitored using the APTT. As with hirudin and bivalirudin, there is no specific reversal agent. Argatroban has been used principally in the management of HIT and during percutaneous coronary procedures in patients at risk of HIT.

Oral direct thrombin inhibitors

Dabigatran

Dabigatran is a synthetic small molecule direct thrombin inhibitor, which binds reversibly to both fibrin-bound and free thrombin. It is administered orally as the pro-drug dabigatran etexilate and is rapidly metabolized to the active drug dabigatran. Bioavailability is low at 4–5 per cent and is further reduced by concomitant use of proton pump inhibitors. Peak concentrations are reached within 2 hours, and the plasma half-life is 14–17 hours, permitting once-daily dosage.

Clearance is predominantly renal, and dose adjustment in renal failure may be necessary. Unlike coumarins, dabigatran clearance is not dependent on the cytochrome P450 enzymes.

Dabigatran does not require routine dose monitoring. Dabigatran causes prolongation of the APTT, but not in a linear dose-dependent fashion—more accurate monitoring can be achieved using the ecarin clotting time. The most common adverse effects are bleeding and an elevation of liver transaminases. The frequency and significance of elevated liver transaminases during dabigatran are yet to be established.

Oral direct factor Xa antagonists

Several oral direct factor Xa antagonists, which do not require antithrombin to exert their activity, are undergoing clinical trials.

Rivaroxaban

Rivaroxaban is a direct inhibitor of factor Xa. It has an oral bioavailability of 60–80 per cent, and has a rapid onset of action, reaching peak concentration at 3 hours. The half-life is 5–9 hours. Excretion is predominantly renal. It is undergoing phase III trials and so far, like dabigatran, has not exhibited any major side effects in orthopaedic surgery as well as has a good efficacy profile.[32]

Apixaban

Apixaban is also an orally bioavailable small molecule direct factor Xa inhibitor. Bioavailability is 50–85 per cent, peak concentration is reached at 3 hours, and the half-life is 9–14 hours. It is undergoing phase III trials. Excretion is predominantly biliary and so it may be useful in renal failure.[33]

There are a number of other novel oral anticoagulants in the pipeline, thus suggesting that the days of widespread warfarin and heparin usage are numbered.[34]

Considerations in patients with advanced disease

We have attempted to illustrate specific issues in the palliative setting that may influence the choice, dosage, or monitoring of anticoagulants throughout the chapter as they have arisen. The most pertinent factors that should be considered are outlined below.

Variable oral absorption

Warfarin and other coumarins have high oral bioavailability of nearly 100 per cent. Successful anticoagulation can be achieved even when gut transit time is short or in patients with short bowel syndrome. The anticoagulant activity of warfarin may be in fact increased in patients with abnormal oral absorption due to reduced vitamin K absorption (particularly in those with cholestasis), or to protein malnutrition and consequent hypoalbuminaemia. Close therapeutic drug monitoring is recommended.

Nausea and vomiting may be a greater problem, as warfarin is administered once daily. In patients with frequent vomiting, a parenteral anticoagulant such as subcutaneous LMWH may be more appropriate.

Variable absorption may prove a significant issue with some of the newer oral anticoagulants. Dabigatran, in particular, has a low oral bioavailability of around 5 per cent, and may require therapeutic monitoring in those with rapid intestinal transit times or short bowel.

Anticoagulants, which are dosed according to weight such as treatment doses of LMWH may require intermittent dose adjustment in patients with weight loss.

Hypoalbuminaemia

Whether due to malnutrition, the acute phase response, or to a renal or intestinal protein losing-state, hypoalbuminaemia is common in palliative care. Coumarins such as warfarin are >99 per cent bound to plasma proteins, predominantly to albumin. Hypoalbuminaemia results in an increased proportion of free warfarin, increased anticoagulant activity, and potentially an increased bleeding risk. Warfarin requires closer therapeutic monitoring in those with hypoalbuminaemia, and use of an alternative anticoagulant carrying lower bleeding risk is preferable.

Drug interactions

The use of multiple and changing medications in palliative care can significantly affect the dose requirements for coumarins. All coumarins are metabolized by cytochrome P450 enzymes, which are induced or inhibited by a wide range of drugs, foods, and herbal remedies. Antibiotic, antifungal, and antiepileptic medications are particularly implicated, but numerous other medications can also interact with coumarins.

LMWH do not have extensive drug interactions, and may be more appropriate in palliative care patients who require multiple medications.

Chemo- and radiotherapy

Anticoagulation during chemo- or radiotherapy can pose specific problems. Nausea, vomiting, and diarrhoea may affect intestinal absorption of oral anticoagulants and of vitamin K. Weight loss and hypoalbuminaemia may necessitate dose adjustment. Thrombocytopenia due to marrow suppression may cause an increase in bleeding risk.

In general, parenteral anticoagulants such as LMWH or fondaparinux are preferable to coumarins during chemo- or radiotherapy. During periods of severe thrombocytopenia (platelets $<20 \times 10^9$ per L), the anticoagulant can be temporarily omitted until the platelet count recovers. If oral vitamin K antagonists are to be used, the frequency of therapeutic monitoring should be increased.

Quality of life

In patients with advanced disease, clinical decision-making must take into consideration the impact the available treatments have on quality of life. For some, the treatment and possible complications of therapies may be more distressing than the symptoms of the condition itself. There is limited qualitative data on the impact of anticoagulants in the primary and secondary thromboprophylaxis of VTE in the palliative care setting.[21,35] These papers suggest that LMWH is an acceptable intervention in the advanced cancer population and that the repeated venepunctures required for monitiong of warfarin safely had a negative impact. However, the applicability of this data across all patients with advanced disease is open to debate, and the views of each individual are likely to vary.

Key points

- ◆ LMWH are the mainstay of prophylactic and therapeutic anticoagulation for VTE in palliative care and do not require routine therapeutic monitoring. Dose adjustment is required in renal failure and weight loss.

- ◆ Danaparoid or the synthetic pentasaccharides fondaparinux and idraparinux can be used as alternatives to LMWH for thromboprophylaxis and treatment of VTE, and are safe in patients with a history of HIT. Dose adjustment is required in renal failure.

- ◆ UFH is useful in those with renal failure, but platelet count should be monitored because of the risk of HIT. Treatment dose UFH requires therapeutic drug monitoring.

- ◆ Oral vitamin K antagonists are suitable for the long-term anticoagulation of clinically stable patients. Because of their long duration of action, narrow therapeutic index and myriad of drug and food interactions control may be problematic in the palliative care setting. Conversion to LMWH should be considered in advanced cancer, during chemo- or radiotherapy, where interactions prove problematic, where therapeutic drug monitoring is impractical or unacceptable, or where a stable INR cannot be achieved.

- ◆ Parenteral direct thrombin inhibitors such as hirudins, argatroban, and bivalirudin are useful in the management of HIT, but the requirement for close therapeutic drug monitoring limits their use.

- ◆ Oral direct thrombin inhibitors such as dabigatran and oral factor Xa antagonists such as rivaroxaban and apixaban are currently in clinical trials. These may provide effective anticoagulation without the need for routine therapeutic monitoring. The use of these agents may become widespread.

Selected case scenarios highlighting difficult clinical scenarios

Case 1: renal failure

A 70-year-old male with severe cardiac failure and end-stage renal failure requiring peritoneal dialysis presented with a left ventricular mural thrombosis.

He was anticoagulated with intravenous UFH at therapeutic doses, aiming for a target APTT-R of 1.5–2.5 (the local reference range). Venous access proved problematic, so he was switched to subcutaneous UFH at 250 IU/kg 12-hourly. APTT-R was checked 4–6 hours post-dose, and the subcutaneous UFH dose adjusted to achieve the target range. Platelet count was checked on alternate days whilst on heparin to monitor for HIT.

Once clinically stable, warfarin was commenced aiming for a target INR of 2.0–3.0 long term. UFH was stopped once the INR was therapeutic for 2 consecutive days.

LMWH should be avoided, or anti-Xa activity monitoring instituted, in patients with end-stage renal failure as accumulation with consequent bleeding can occur. UFH and warfarin are both suitable in renal failure. Intravenous UFH can present practical difficulties due to the need for continuous intravenous access and frequent blood tests. Subcutaneous UFH can be administered at therapeutic doses, and may circumvent some of these difficulties.

Case 2: heparin-induced thrombocytopenia

A 68-year-old smoker with type 2 diabetes mellitus and hyperlipidaemia had a strong history of arterial vascular disease including myocardial infarction, ischaemic cerebrovascular accident, and claudication due to peripheral vascular disease. He presented with an ischaemic left leg. Intravenous UFH was commenced with a 5,000 IU bolus followed by an infusion starting at 1,400 IU/h and adjusted according to APTT-R. He underwent surgical embolectomy, leading to a resolution of his ischaemia. Subsequently, he developed a compartment syndrome in his left calf as a consequence of reperfusion injury. This required surgical fasciotomy. Intravenous UFH was continued, having been stopped 2 hours before surgery and resumed afterwards.

The platelet count began to fall on the fifth day, and on the eighth day the patient had a platelet count of 70×10^9/L. The admission platelet count had been 240×10^9/L. He was considered at high risk of having HIT in view of the significant fall in platelet count, the consistent timing, and the lack of another cause of thrombocytopenia. Pending the results of laboratory tests for HIT, heparin was stopped, and an intravenous infusion of hirudins commenced and adjusted to achieve a target APTT-R of 2.0–2.5.

The platelet count began to rise after 2 days of hirudin, and after 5 days had normalized. ELISA and platelet aggregation studies were positive for HIT. The patient was loaded with warfarin, and hirudin stopped after the INR was therapeutic for 2 consecutive days. He was advised that he had had HIT and was issued an 'allergy card' detailing his adverse reaction.

HIT occurs in 0.3–6.5 per cent of those receiving UFH. It can also occur in patients treated with LMWH. HIT should be suspected when patients receiving heparins have a fall in platelet count of 50 per cent compared to baseline starting between 5 and 10 days after heparin initiation. Arterial and venous thromboses may occur. Clinical risk stratification scores are useful.

If there is a strong suspicion of HIT, appropriate treatment should be started pending the results of confirmatory tests. All heparins should be stopped and an alternative anticoagulant such as hirudin, danaparoid, or fondaparinux commenced. Coumarins should not be started in acute HIT until the patient is fully anticoagulated with another drug.

Once the platelet count has normalized, anticoagulants can be stopped unless there is a need for ongoing anticoagulation. Patients should be informed of their diagnosis and advised to avoid UFH in the future. Re-exposure to short duration LMWH with close platelet count monitoring may be safe as long as at least 100 days have elapsed since the acute HIT episode.

Case 3: unstable INR

A 52-year-old woman with stage IV diffuse large B-cell lymphoma had bilateral iliac deep vein thromboses at presentation due to extensive pelvic lymphadenopathy. She was anticoagulated with treatment doses of a LMWH, and commenced warfarin loading. LMWH was stopped once her INR had been in the therapeutic range for 2 consecutive days.

Once a histological diagnosis had been established, she commenced chemotherapy with cyclophosphamide, doxorubicin, vincristine, prednisolone, and rituximab (CHOP-R) chemotherapy 3-weekly. Despite weekly therapeutic monitoring, her INR proved unstable during chemotherapy. Factors contributing to the INR instability included chemotherapy-induced anorexia, interactions with co-trimoxazole antibacterial prophylaxis, and a course of fluconazole given for oral candidiasis.

Warfarin was stopped and LMWH recommenced at therapeutic doses. The patient was taught to self-inject this and was provided with a supply of pre-filled LMWH syringes and a sharps bin. Platelet count was monitored during the first 2 weeks of therapy to exclude HIT. Routine platelet count monitoring for LMWH was stopped after this point, as HIT does not occur beyond the first 2 weeks of treatment. LMWH was continued throughout chemotherapy without therapeutic monitoring and without bleeding complications. LMWH was stopped after 3 months, as the patient was in clinical remission and her pelvic lymphadenopathy had resolved.

Numerous factors complicate the use of coumarins during chemotherapy. Anorexia and vomiting, hypoalbuminaemia, and drug interactions contribute to INR instability. LMWH have the advantage of fewer drug interactions, no dependence upon oral absorption or vitamin K status, and no requirement for monitoring. Bleeding and thrombosis risks are also lower. The major disadvantage is the requirement for daily subcutaneous injection, but most patients can be taught to safely self-inject LMWH at home.

Case 4: bleeding whilst on LMWH

A 61-year-old woman with relapsed metastatic small cell carcinoma of the lung presented with a left iliac deep vein thrombosis. Renal function was normal. Treatment dose LMWH (enoxaparin 1.5 mg/kg subcutaneously once daily) was commenced, and the patient was taught to self-inject at home. Warfarin was not initiated because of active malignancy and excessive bleeding risk.

Eight weeks later, she developed haemoptysis with expectoration of approximately 10 mL of fresh blood. She was known to have extensive pulmonary involvement by carcinoma. She was cachectic, her weight having fallen from 68 to 50 kg since starting enoxaparin. Renal function remained normal.

Her enoxaparin dose was reduced from 100 to 75 mg daily according to her new body weight. Palliative radiotherapy was arranged. No further bleeding problems occurred.

In patients with changing body weight, regular review of the anticoagulant dose may be necessary. Bleeding does not always require cessation of anticoagulants. In this case, the risk of further thrombosis without anti-coagulation was judged to be very high so anticoagulation was continued at a reduced dose.

References

1. Marcum JA. The origin of the dispute over the discovery of heparin. *Journal of the History of Medicine and Allied Sciences* 2000;55:37–66.
2. Mulloy B, Gray E, Barrowcliffe TW. Characterisation of unfractionated heparin: comparison of materials from the last 50 years. *Thrombosis and Haemostasis* 2000;84:1052–6.
3. Hirsh J, Raschke R, Warkentin TE *et al.* Heparin: mechanism of action, pharmacokinetics, dosing considerations, monitoring, efficacy, and safety. *Chest* 1995;108:258S–75S.

4. Hommes DW, Bura A, Mazzolai L *et al.* Subcutaneous heparin compared with continuous heparin administration in the initial treatment of deep vein thrombosis. A meta-analysis. *Annals of Internal Medicine* 1992;116:279–84.

5. Kearon C, Ginsberg JS, Julian JA *et al.* Comparison of fixed-dose weight-adjusted unfractionated heparin and low molecular weight heparin for acute treatment of venous thromboembolism. *Journal of the American Medical Association* 2006;296:935–42.

6. Kitchen S, Preston FE. The therapeutic range for heparin therapy: relationship between six activated partial thromboplastin time reagents and two heparin assays. *Thrombosis and Haemostasis* 1996;75:734–9.

7. Hirsh J, Raschke R. Heparin and low-molecular-weight heparin. The Seventh ACCP Conference on Antithrombotic and Thrombolytic Therapy. *Chest* 1994;126:188S–203S.

8. Keeling D, Davidson S, Watson H. The management of heparin-induced thrombocytopenia. *British Journal of Haematology* 2006;133:259–69.

9. Lo GK, Juhl D, Warkentin TE *et al.* Evaluation of pre-test clinical score (4 T's) for the diagnosis of heparin-induced thrombocytopenia in two clinical settings. *Journal of Thrombosis and Haemostasis* 2006;4:759–65.

10. Baglin T, Barrowcliffe TW, Cohen A *et al.* Guidelines on the use and monitoring of heparin. *British Journal of Haematology* 2006;133:19–34.

11. Davidson BL, Büller HR, Decousus H *et al.* Effect of obesity on outcomes after fondaparinux, enoxaparin, or heparin treatment for acute venous thromboembolism in the Matisse trials. *Journal of Thrombosis and Haemostasis* 2007;5:1191–4.

12. Scholten DJ, Hoedema RM, Scholten SE. A comparison of two different prophylactic dose regimens of low molecular weight heparin in bariatric surgery. *Obesity Surgery* 2002;12:19–24.

13. Thorevska N, Amoateng-Adjepong Y, Sabahi R *et al.* Anticoagulation in hospitalized patients with renal insufficiency: a comparison of bleeding rates with unfractionated heparin vs enoxaparin. *Chest* 2004;125:856–63.

14. Martel N, Lee J, Wells PS. Risk for heparin-induced thrombocytopenia with unfractionated and low molecular weight heparin thromboprophylaxis: a meta-analysis. *Blood* 2005;106:2710–5.

15. Morris TA, Castrejon S, Devendra G *et al.* No difference in risk for thrombocytopenia during treatment of pulmonary embolism & deep venous thrombosis with either low molecular weight heparin or unfractionated heparin: a meta-analysis. *Chest* 2007;132:1131–9.

16. Rajgopal R, Bear M, Butcher MK *et al.* The effects of heparin and low molecular weight heparins on bone. *Thrombosis Research* 2008;122(3):293–8.

17. Noble SI, Hood K, Finlay IG. The use of long-term low-molecular weight heparin for the treatment of venous thromboembolism in palliative care patients with advanced cancer: a case series of sixty two patients. *Palliative Medicine* 2007;21:473–6

18. Ludwig RJ, Schindewolf M, Alban S *et al.* Molecular weight determines the frequency of delayed type hypersensitivity reactions to heparin and synthetic oligosaccharides. *Thrombosis and Haemostasis* 2005;94:1265–9.

19. Laposata M, Green D, Van Cott EM *et al.* College of American Pathologists Conference XXXI on laboratory monitoring of anticoagulant therapy. The clinical use and laboratory monitoring of low molecular weight heparin, danaparoid, hirudin, and related compounds, and argatroban. *Archives of Pathology and Laboratory Medicine* 1998;122:799–807.

20. Mueller RL, Scheidt S. History of drugs for thrombotic disease. Discovery, development, and directions for the future. *Circulation* 1994;89:432–49.

21. Noble SI, Finlay IG. Is long-term low-molecular-weight heparin acceptable to palliative care patients in the treatment of cancer related venous thromboembolism? A qualitative study. *Palliative Medicine* 2005;19:197–201.

22. Baglin TP, Keeling DM, Watson HG. Guidelines on oral anticoagulation (warfarin): third edition – 2005 update. *British Journal of Haematology* 2005;132:277–85.

23. Johnson MJ. Problems of anticoagulation within a palliative care setting: an audit of hospice patients taking warfarin. *Palliative Medicine* 1997;11:306–12.

24. Palareti G, Leali N, Coccheri S *et al.* Bleeding complications of oral anticoagulant treatment: an inception-cohort, prospective collaborative study (ISCOAT). *Lancet* 1996;348:423–8.

25. Kuderer NM, Khorana AA, Lyman GH *et al.* A meta-analysis and systematic review of the efficacy and safety of anticoagulants as cancer treatment: impact on survival and bleeding complications. *Cancer* 2007;110:1149–61.

26. Prandoni P, Lensing AW, Piccioli A *et al.* Recurrent venous thromboembolism and bleeding complications during anticoagulant treatment in patients with cancer and venous thrombosis. *Blood* 2002;100:3484–8.

27. Lee AY, Levine MN, Baker RI *et al.* Low-molecular-weight heparin versus a coumarin for the prevention of recurrent venous thromboembolism in patients with cancer. *New England Journal of Medicine* 2003;349:146–53.

28. Young G, Yonekawa KE, Nakagawa PA *et al.* Recombinant activated factor VII effectively reverses the anticoagulant effects of heparin, enoxaparin, fondparinux, argatroban, and bivalirudin ex vivo as measured using thromboelastography. *Blood Coagulation and Fibrinolysis* 2007;18:547–53.

29. Van Gogh Investigators, Buller HR, Cohen AT *et al.* Idraparinux versus standard therapy for venous thromboembolic disease. *New England Journal of Medicine* 2007;357:1094–104.

30. Van Gogh Investigators, Buller HR, Cohen AT *et al.* Extended prophylaxis of venous thromboembolism with idraparinux. *New England Journal of Medicine* 2007;357:1105–12.

31. Eichler P, Friesen H, Lubenow N *et al.* Antihirudin antibodies in patients with heparin-induced thrombocytopenia treated with lepirudin: incidence, effects on aPTT, and clinical relevance. *Blood* 2000;96:2373–8.

32. Fisher WD, Eriksson BI, Bauer KA *et al.* Rivaroxaban for thromboprophylaxis after orthopaedic surgery: pooled analysis of two studies. *Thrombosis and Haemostasis* 2007;97:931–7.

33. Weitz JI. Emerging anticoagulants for the treatment of venous thromboembolism. *Thrombosis and Haemostasis* 2006;96:274–84.

34. Hirsh J, O'Donnell M, Eikelboom JW. Beyond unfractionated heparin and warfarin: current and future advances. *Circulation* 2007;116:552–60.

35. Noble SI, Nelson A, Turner C *et al.* Acceptability of low molecular weight heparin thromboprophylaxis for inpatients receiving palliative care: qualitative study. *British Medical Journal* 2006;332:577–80.

Chapter 6

Treatment and secondary prevention of venous thromboembolism in advanced cancer

Agnes Y.Y. Lee

Introduction

Approximately 20 per cent of all cases of venous thromboembolism (VTE) are related to underlying malignancy. Many of these patients have advanced disease or are receiving cancer-directed therapy with the aim of palliation rather than cure. Consequently, physicians are frequently faced with the challenging task of managing VTE in patients with high risks of recurrent thrombosis and serious bleeding, in whom standard anticoagulant therapy may not be the most appropriate treatment. Furthermore, given the short life expectancy of many of these patients,[1,2] quality of life is a particularly important consideration in management planning. Solid evidence from randomized clinical trials have shown that low molecular weight heparin (LMWH) is more efficacious than traditional vitamin K antagonist therapy for secondary prevention of VTE, and provocative clinical data have emerged to suggest that LMWHs may improve cancer patient survival.[3–6] However, many aspects of treatment, such as duration of therapy, remain unstudied. This chapter will review the general approach to treating cancer patients with acute deep vein thrombosis (DVT) or pulmonary embolism (PE) and briefly discuss some controversial areas of management. Several case scenarios with difficult clinical issues are included at the end to further illustrate management options and considerations that are unique to patients with advanced disease.

Initial therapy of VTE

The traditional regimen for the treatment of acute VTE consists of initial therapy with unfractionated heparin (UFH) or LMWH followed by long-term therapy with a vitamin K antagonist, such as warfarin and acenocoumarol, to prevent recurrent thrombosis. This two-phase approach is largely a result of the delayed onset of action of vitamin K antagonists and the resultant need to administer another agent that can achieve a rapid anticoagulant effect. Consequently, the use of a single anticoagulant with a rapid onset of action that is also safe and well tolerated when administered over an extended period of time can simplify therapy.

Choice of anticoagulants

The traditional anticoagulants for the initial treatment of acute VTE are UFH and LMWH. In addition, fondaparinux, a pentasaccharide with indirect inhibitory activity against activated factor X, recently became available in some countries for the initial treatment of VTE,[7,8] and idraparinux, a long-acting derivative of fondaparinux, has been evaluated for long-term treatment.[9,10] According to a Cochrane Database of Systematic Reviews published in 2004, a meta-analysis of 22 randomized trials found that subcutaneous LMWH is more effective than intravenous UFH, and significantly reduces the occurrence of major hemorrhage during initial treatment and overall mortality at follow-up.[11] Furthermore, LMWH can be given once daily in an outpatient setting, without the need for laboratory monitoring, and has a lower risk of heparin-induced thrombocytopenia.[12] A recent randomized trial showed that UFH can be given subcutaneously using weight-based dosage, but twice-daily, large volume injections are required.[13] In many developed countries, outpatient LMWH is considered the standard of care for the initial treatment in patients with DVT or hemodynamically stable PE.

However, whether LMWH, UFH, and fondaparinux are equally effective and safe in patients with cancer has not been formally investigated. Patients with advanced disease or significant comorbid conditions were generally excluded from participation in clinical trials that tested these agents. Based on published data extracted from trials that reported on the outcomes of the subgroup of cancer patients, it appears that weight-adjusted, subcutaneous doses of LMWH and activated partial thromboplastin time- (APTT-) adjusted intravenous infusions of UFH have similar efficacy in patients with and without cancer (Table 6.1).[14–17] Data on the bleeding risk of therapeutic doses of these anticoagulants in cancer patients have not been published. Nonetheless, it is reasonable to assume that UFH and LMWH are comparable in their efficacy in preventing recurrent VTE and in their risk of major hemorrhage in most patients with advanced disease. The experience with fondaparinux and idraparinux in cancer patients has not been published.

On a practical comparison, LMWH remains more attractive than UFH because outpatient LMWH therapy eliminates the need for routine hospitalization

Table 6.1 The efficacy of LMWH and UFH for initial therapy of VTE in patients with and without cancer.

		3-month incidence of symptomatic recurrent VTE		
	No. of patients	LMWH (per cent)	UFH (per cent)	P-value
Cancer	546	9.2	9.2	NS
No cancer	2275	4.0	4.2	NS

Note: combined results from 4 randomized trials showing the 3-month rates of recurrent VTE separately for patients with and without cancer.[14–17]

and requires only once-daily injections. LMWH also comes in precalibrated, prefilled syringes, which reduces the risk of dosing errors compared with having to draw up UFH from multi-dose vials. These are important advantages for patients and their families. Cohort studies have shown that cancer patients can be treated safely at home with LMWH.[18–21] The vast majority of patients are able to perform self-injections when they are given adequate support and appropriate education. For patients who do require hospitalization to control severe symptoms or receive additional supportive therapy, LMWH may still be more attractive than UFH because it requires less nursing time, obviates the need for drawing blood samples for monitoring the anticoagulant effect, and reduces drug dosing errors. Cost-minimization modeling has also shown that LMWH is less expensive than UFH for the inpatient treatment of DVT among cancer patients.[22]

New oral anticoagulants are in advanced stages of development and these may replace parenteral agents for the initial treatment of VTE. However, clinical trials specifically designed to study these novel agents in cancer patients are not yet planned. Such trials are needed to specifically address the more aggressive natural history of VTE and the higher likelihood of drug interactions, organ dysfunction, and bleeding in patients with cancer.

Once- or twice-daily dosing of LMWH

For initial treatment, subcutaneous LMWH may be administered either once daily or twice daily and some agents have regulatory approval for both regimens. Significant differences in efficacy and safety between these regimens have not been shown, although some studies have suggested that twice-daily injection may be more efficacious.[17,23] Given the hypercoagulable status of cancer patients, it might be worth considering switching to twice-daily injections in patients who develop recurrent VTE while receiving therapeutic doses of once-daily LMWH, because twice-daily administration might provide a more steady state of anticoagulation. This hypothesis, however, has not been properly tested. Some also argue that twice-daily dosing may reduce the risk of bleeding by avoiding high peak plasma levels. This theoretical benefit also has not been demonstrated in the clinical setting. Given current evidence available, once-daily injection of LMWH is an acceptable standard of practice.

Long-term therapy

Vitamin K antagonists

Vitamin K antagonists are the mainstay of long-term anticoagulant treatment for preventing recurrent VTE and warfarin is the most commonly used agent worldwide.[12] Warfarin is administered along with a heparin or fondaparinux and is continued for a minimum of 3 months. Owing to differences in the anticoagulant response between and within patients over time, dose adjustments are needed based on the achieved anticoagulant effect, as measured by the international normalized ratio (INR). For the treatment of VTE, the target therapeutic INR range is 2.0–3.0. When vitamin K antagonist therapy is used following therapeutic doses of UFH, LMWH, or fondaparinux, the 3-month risk of symptomatic recurrent VTE is approximately 3–4 per cent for most patients.

But in patients with cancer, vitamin K antagonist therapy is problematic. Owing to its pharmacology, unpredictable anticoagulant responses can result from drug interactions, changes in vitamin K status, liver dysfunction, and gastrointestinal disturbances such as vomiting and diarrhea. Furthermore, because vitamin K antagonists have a delayed onset of action and prolonged clearance of the anticoagulant effect, they are difficult to manage in patients who require repeat invasive procedures (e.g., therapeutic paracentesis, spinal taps) or experience frequent episodes of chemotherapy-induced thrombocytopenia.

Cancer patients treated with warfarin also experience frequent recurrent VTE and have a high risk of major bleeding. According to prospective studies, the annual risk of recurrent VTE is 21–27 per cent in cancer patients while on warfarin therapy.[24,25] This is 2- to 3-fold higher than in patients without cancer. Recurrent VTE can also occur when the INR is therapeutic (Table 6.2).[25] Cancer patients on oral anticoagulant therapy also have an annual risk of major bleeding of 12–13 per cent, versus 3–4 per cent for patients without cancer (Table 6.2).[24,25] In contrast to patients without cancer, the risk of bleeding in cancer patients does not correlate with the INR level and it continues to increase over the course of therapy.

Table 6.2 The incidence of recurrent VTE and major bleeding in relation to the INR.[25]

INR range	Cancer No. of events (per 100 pt-years)	No cancer No. of events (per 100 pt-years)	Total No. of events (per 100 pt-years)
Recurrent VTE			
≤ 2.0	54.0	15.9	23.7
2.1–3.0	18.9	7.2	9.2
> 3.0	18.4	6.4	8.7
Major bleeding			
≤ 2.0	30.6	0.0	3.1
2.1–3.0	11.2	0.8	2.6
> 3.0	0.0	6.3	5.1

LMWH

In contrast to vitamin K antagonists, LMWH does not require routine laboratory monitoring and has minimal drug interactions. The parenteral route of administration also ensures drug delivery, especially in patients who are unable to tolerate oral intake or have significant gastrointestinal problems. Finally, dose adjustments or withholding of LMWH can be made readily to accommodate thrombocytopenia or invasive procedures. However, LMWH should be used with caution in patients with renal dysfunction and is associated with a low risk of heparin-induced thrombocytopenia and a marginal reduction in bone mineral density.[26,27] Given the short life expectancy of most patients with cancer and thrombosis, osteopenia or osteoporosis are not relevant concerns.

To date, a number of open-label trials have compared different LMWHs with vitamin K antagonists for the long-term treatment of VTE (Table 6.3). The CANTHANOX trial compared 3 months of standard warfarin therapy with enoxaparin in cancer patients with proximal DVT, PE or both.[28] Only 147 patients were randomized and the study was closed prematurely because of slow recruitment. After 3 months of treatment, 15 of 71 patients in the warfarin group had recurrent VTE or major bleeding, as compared with 7 of 67 patients assigned to receive enoxaparin (P=0.09). There were six fatal bleeding events in patients receiving warfarin and none in the enoxaparin group. Another study evaluating two different doses of enoxaparin for long-term treatment showed that patients were compliant with self-injections, but the study was underpowered to demonstrate any difference between warfarin and enoxaparin regimens.[29]

Table 6.3 Randomized controlled trials evaluating monotherapy with LMWH for long-term treatment of VTE in cancer patients.

Study	N*	Treatment regimens	Recurrent VTE during treatment (per cent)	Major bleeding during treatment (per cent)	Death (per cent)	P-value for primary outcome
Meyer[28]	71	Initial: enoxaparin (1.5 mg/kg OD for ≥4 days)	21.1		22.7	0.09[1]
	67	Long-term: warfarin (INR 2–3 for 3 months) Enoxaparin (1.5 mg/kg OD for 3 months)	10.5		11.3	
Lee[30]	336	Initial: dalteparin (200 IU/kg for 5–7 days)	17	4	41	0.002[2]
	336	Long-term: coumarin (INR 2–3 for 6 months) Dalteparin (200 IU/kg OD for 1 month) then Dalteparin (~150 IU/kg OD for 5 months)	9	6	39	
Deitcher[29]	30	Initial: enoxparin (1 mg/kg BID for 5 days) Long-term: warfarin (INR 2–3 for 180 days)	10.0	2.9	8.8	NS[3]
	29	Initial: enoxaparin (1 mg/kg BID for 5 days) Long-term: enoxaparin(1 mg/kg OD for 175 days)	6.9	6.5	6.5	
	32	Initial: enoxaparin (1 mg/kg BID for 5 days) Long-term: enoxaparin (1.5 mg/kg OD for 175 days)	6.3	11.1	19.4	
Hull[32]	100	Initial: IV UFH (APTT adjusted for 6 days)	10	7	19	NS[4]
	100	Long-term: warfarin (INR 2–3 for 3 months) Tinzaparin (175 IU/kg OD for 3 months)	6	7	20	

* N, denotes number of patients evaluable for the primary outcome in the respective treatment groups. NS, not statistically significant.
[1] Primary outcome was a composite endpoint of objectively documented recurrent VTE or major bleeding. There was no statistically significant difference between treatment groups with a relative risk of 2.02 (95 per cent confidence interval [CI] 0.88–4.65).
[2] Primary outcome of cumulative incidence of objectively, documented recurrent VTE was assessed at 6 months. Hazard ratio in the dalteparin group as compared with the coumarin group was 0.48 (95 per cent CI 0.30–0.77), log-rank P=0.002.
[3] Primary objective was to evaluate the feasibility of recruitment and compliance with long-term (180 days) injections of enoxaparin. No difference was observed in overall compliance with an average rate of 95 per cent amongst all groups.
[4] Primary outcome measure of objectively, documented recurrent VTE or death was assessed at 3 months. There was no statistically significant difference between treatment groups (difference –4.0 [95 per cent CI 12.0–4.1]).

The CLOT trial randomized 676 cancer patients with acute VTE to usual treatment with dalteparin followed by vitamin K antagonist therapy or dalteparin alone for 6 months.[30] In the dalteparin group, patients received therapeutic doses at 200 IU per kg once daily for the first month and then 75–80 per cent of the full dose for the next 5 months. In the control group, patients received therapeutic doses of dalteparin for a minimum of 5 days and a vitamin K antagonist at doses to target the INR values at 2.5 for 6 months. All patients were followed-up for symptomatic recurrent VTE, bleeding, and death. These outcomes were centrally adjudicated by an expert committee masked to treatment assignment. Over the 6-month treatment period, 27 of 338 in the dalteparin group and 53 of 338 in the vitamin K antagonist group had symptomatic, recurrent VTE. The cumulative risk of recurrent VTE was reduced from 17 per cent in the vitamin K antagonist group to 9 per cent in the dalteparin group, resulting in a statistically significant risk reduction of 52 per cent (P=0.002). The INR values were therapeutic or higher during 70 per cent of the total treatment time, indicating that patients in the control group were adequately treated. Accordingly, one episode of recurrent VTE is prevented for every 13 patients treated with dalteparin. Overall, there were no differences in major or any bleeding; 6 per cent of patients in the dalteparin group versus 4 per cent of the control group experienced major bleeding. By 6 months, about 40 per cent of the patients in each group had died; 90 per cent were due to progressive cancer. Following the CLOT trial, a prospective cohort study evaluated whether a fixed dose of dalteparin once daily is effective and safe for long-term treatment. The study included 203 patients with metastatic cancer who received an initial 7-day course of weight-adjusted dalteparin followed by dalteparin 10,000 IU once daily, regardless of the patient's weight. During the 3-month follow-up period, 18 patients (9 per cent) developed recurrent VTE and 11 patients (5 per cent) had major bleeding.[31]

Lastly, a smaller randomized trial compared tinzaparin with warfarin for long-term use in cancer patients.[32] In this study, 100 patients were randomized to receive 3 months of tinzaparin 175 IU per kg once daily and 100 were assigned to receive usual care with intravenous UFH and warfarin. At the end of the 3-month treatment period, 6 per cent of patients in the tinzaparin group versus 10 per cent of the usual care group had developed symptomatic recurrent VTE. This difference was not statistically significant (−4.0 per cent; 95 per cent CI, 12.0–4.1 per cent). Both groups had similar incidences of major bleeding and overall mortality.

Based on the above evidence, LMWH is recommended for extended treatment in cancer patients by the 2004 American College of Chest Physicians

Consensus Guidelines,[12] the British Society of Haematology,[33] the Italian Association of Medical Oncology,[34] the National Comprehensive Cancer Network,[35] and the American Society of Clinical Oncology guideline[36] as the treatment of choice for cancer patients with VTE. Currently, dalteparin is the only LMWH to receive regulatory approval for the extended treatment of VTE in patients with cancer.

Pentasaccharides

The long-acting pentasaccharide idraparinux has been evaluated as an alternative to vitamin K antagonist therapy. In a multicentre study, 1,215 patients were randomized to receive idraparinux 2.5 mg or placebo subcutaneous injections once weekly after completing 6 months of therapy with an anticoagulant.(10) After 6 months of study treatment, 1.0 per cent of patients in the idraparinux group versus 3.7 per cent in the placebo group had recurrent VTE (P=0.002), while 1.9 per cent versus none had major bleeding, respectively (P<0.001). There were 120 patients with cancer in the study but their results were not reported separately. Given the increased risk of bleeding, the lack of a specific antidote, and the prolonged duration of anticoagulant effects, idraparinux does not appear to be suitable or practical in cancer patients.

Duration of therapy

The length of treatment with an anticoagulant for the secondary prevention of recurrent VTE has not been well studied in patients with cancer or advanced disease. These patients are usually excluded from clinical trials studying optimal duration, and their high risk of bleeding and other medical complications make continuation of anticoagulation challenging. Therefore, it may not be appropriate to extrapolate the results from available clinical trials and apply them to patients with advanced disease.

In general, a minimum of 3–6 months of treatment is prescribed. Beyond this period, based on the consensus that patients with ongoing or irreversible risk factors for VTE need an extended duration of anticoagulant therapy, 'indefinite' therapy is traditionally recommended in patients with metastatic disease. In a recent study in 62 patients with advanced, metastatic cancer and VTE, three of the seven patients who stopped LMWH after 6 months of treatment developed symptomatic, recurrent thrombosis.[37] Two other studies reported recurrence of VTE in 13 per cent and 42 per cent of patients with advanced cancer after cessation of anticoagulant therapy.[38,39] In patients without metastases, anticoagulant treatment is indicated while the cancer is 'active'. This usually means that anticoagulation is continued if cancer is clinically detectable or while the patient is receiving antitumor therapy.

Patients should be re-evaluated frequently to assess the risk–benefit ratio of continuing anticoagulant therapy. Besides the risks of recurrence and bleeding, the patient's quality of life, life expectancy, and personal preference should be taken into strong consideration. Without evidence from randomized trials or validated methods of identifying patients who would benefit from extended secondary prevention, anticoagulant therapy beyond the usual 6-month period must be carefully assessed and tailored to the needs and preference of each individual patient.

Treatment in patients with recurrent VTE or bleeding

Treatment of recurrent VTE

LMWH has been shown in small case series to be effective in treating patients who develop recurrent VTE while on warfarin therapy[40] but published data are not available for managing patients who develop recurrence while on LMWH. Feasible approaches include increasing the dose of LMWH, changing to twice-daily injections, or switching to intravenous or subcutaneous UFH. From a convenience point of view, increasing the dose of LMWH is the most attractive and logical option. The anti-factor Xa level may be useful to guide dose increases in such cases. For once-daily dosing, the target anti-Xa level should be approximately 1.0–1.5 U/mL. Anecdotally, patients who breakthrough the standard weight-adjusted doses of LMWH tend to have subtherapeutic antifactor Xa levels and can tolerate dose escalation without experiencing bleeding.

Another option that is often recommended in patients with recurrent VTE is insertion of an inferior vena cava (IVC) filter. However, the indications, efficacy, and safety of this therapeutic modality are poorly studied. In the only randomized trial studying patients with proximal DVT, it was shown that an IVC filter in combination with therapeutic anticoagulant therapy can reduce the risk of PE compared with anticoagulation alone, but patients with filters also had a higher incidence of recurrent DVT (20.8 per cent vs. 11.6 per cent) at 2 years of follow-up.[41] Furthermore, there were no differences in symptomatic PE at 3 months, 1 year, and 2 years. At 8 years of follow-up, there were no differences in recurrent VTE or overall survival between the filter and non-filter groups.[42] A large population-based study also failed to find a significant reduction in the incidence of re-hospitalization for PE in patients following IVC filter insertion.[43] A review examining data from 6490 patients in 88 published case series and one randomized trial reported that PE occurred in 2.6–3.8 per cent, DVT in 6–32 per cent, and IVC thrombosis in 3.6–11.1 per cent of patients after IVC filter insertion.[44]

Overall, published evidence has established that an IVC filter does not provide additional benefit to anticoagulation to general patients with proximal DVT. However, the role of IVC filters in the management of VTE remains unclear.

Evidence for filter use in the oncology population is even weaker. Publications are largely from retrospective or anecdotal experience.[45–49] In one retrospective study, 32 per cent of cancer patients with VTE and IVC filters developed recurrent DVT.[46] It is possible that filters enhance the risk of recurrent DVT because of the heightened hypercoagulable state in cancer patients. In another retrospective study of 116 patients with cancer and filter placement, survival rates were 69 per cent at 30 days, 49 per cent at 3 months, and 27 per cent at 1 year.[49] But clearly, patient selection for filter insertion can bias these results.

Overall, given that there is no evidence that these invasive devices alleviate symptoms of VTE, reduce recurrent VTE or improve overall survival compared with anticoagulant therapy, the use of vena caval filters should be avoided in patients with recurrent VTE who can tolerate anticoagulant therapy. Dose escalation of LMWH is the most feasible and sensible approach to ameliorate symptoms of VTE and prevent further recurrence. It is particularly important to remember that in patients with advanced disease who are receiving end-of-life care, the most important goal of therapy is to maximize symptomatic control and minimize discomfort.

Treatment of VTE in patients with bleeding

Treatment of DVT in patients with active bleeding is particularly challenging and there is no published evidence to guide management. It is essential to discuss the risks and benefits of the available options and individualized management.

Anticoagulant therapy is generally contraindicated in patients with bleeding. However, minor or nuisance bleeding in patients with cancer should not prevent the use of anticoagulants, especially in patients with symptomatic proximal DVT or PE involving segmental or more central pulmonary arteries. In all cases, the first step is to take appropriate measures to stop and treat the source of bleeding, if possible.

In cases where the bleeding can be easily monitored and is arising from a source that is not likely to be life-threatening (e.g., epistaxis), full dose LMWH therapy can be started (or continued) and the patient should be followed-up closely. If the bleeding is from a mucosal surface due to tumor invasion (e.g., bladder carcinoma), more caution is required. In such situations, anticoagulant therapy can be started using prophylactic or subtherapeutic doses. If the severity of bleeding does not worsen and the hemoglobin remains stable, then the dose of LMWH can be slowly increased toward therapeutic levels.

For active bleeding of a more aggressive nature (e.g., intracranial bleed, upper gastrointestinal bleeding) anticoagulant therapy is not recommended. In these cases, an IVC filter may be indicated if the patient has proximal DVT. Permanent filters are preferred over retrievable filters if the bleeding is arising from a critical site as the likelihood of reintroducing anticoagulants is low. Retrievable filters can be used in situations when the risk of thrombus embolization is high and only temporary cessation of anticoagulant therapy is needed (e.g., surgery). These filters can then be removed when hemostasis is achieved. It should be noted that there is no evidence that filter placement will improve the clinical outcome or prognosis of patients with VTE and bleeding. Nonetheless, the use of filters in patients with active, serious bleeding is generally accepted. It is possible that a filter would only increase the risk of DVT extension and worsen symptoms, because it does not suppress the underlying hypercoagulable state. Also, fatal PE can result from thrombus formation in the vena cava proximal to the filter, and this complication has been reported in cancer patients.

Antineoplastic potential of LMWH

In the palliative setting, whether LMWH or other anticoagulants provide a survival benefit is of minimal relevance. However, it is worth noting that experimental studies and clinical trials have shown that LMWH use is associated with a reduction in mortality, particularly in patients with limited or early stage malignancy.[3–6,50] The most compelling evidence comes from two clinical trials. In the MALT study, 302 patients with noncurable solid tumors were randomized to receive nadroparin or placebo for 6 weeks.[5] A statistically significant improvement in median survival was associated with nadroparin. In the Turkish study, 84 patients with newly diagnosed small-cell lung cancer were randomized to receive standard chemotherapy with or without dalteparin.[3] Progression-free survival and overall survival were better in patients who received dalteparin. It is interesting to note that the improvement in survival occurred following the cessation of LMWH therapy in these studies, suggesting that the reason or mechanism for improved survival is not due to a reduction in fatal PE. Although these results need to be confirmed in larger studies and in different tumor types, they do support the concept that activation of coagulation is intrinsically involved in tumor growth and that

LMWH is able to interrupt these critical processes. The exact mechanisms, however, have not been elucidated.

Quality of life

Few studies have addressed quality of life in patients receiving long-term anti-coagulation.[51,52] A qualitative study interviewed 40 palliative care patients who were receiving LMWH for VTE treatment found that patients preferred LMWH over warfarin, which was reported to have a negative impact on quality of life.[51] In contrast to expectations, patients were not distressed by daily injections and did not perceive this as an added burden. Instead, patients reported that LMWH was simpler to administer, provided them freedom from laboratory testing, hospitals, and even worry. A substudy in a randomized trial found that postphlebitic syndrome and ulcer formation occur less frequently in patients treated with LMWH than warfarin therapy.[53]

In patients receiving end-of-life care, it is imperative that the patient and family members are informed of the risks and benefits of starting or continuing anticoagulant therapy. In such patients, the main goal of therapy is to provide symptomatic relief. Hence, it is of questionable benefit to administer anticoagulants in such patients who are asymptomatic from their DVT or PE. More aggressive interventions, such as insertion of an IVC filter, are strongly discouraged in this setting.

Case scenarios

The following cases are designed to illustrate some of the difficult VTE management issues in patients with advanced disease. The therapeutic approaches are based largely on anecdotal experience and are not considered 'standards of practice' or the only options in similar clinical settings.

Case 1: patient with active bleeding and newly diagnosed DVT

A 51-year-old woman presents with swelling in her left leg for 2 weeks. There is no associated pain or discoloration. She does not recall any trauma to the leg and has no obvious risk factors for DVT. She has a history of colon cancer and underwent curative resection 4 years ago. She has had moderate amounts of vaginal bleeding. She attributes this to perimenopausal spotting.

The abdominal examination reveals fullness in the left lower quadrant. Her left leg is swollen and there is tenderness to palpation along the venous distribution. Her left calf circumference measures 39 cm and the right one measures 35 cm. There is pitting edema isolated in her left leg. A pelvic examination reveals an erosive lesion on the left vaginal wall.

A compression B-mode ultrasound showed noncompressibility of the common femoral, superficial, and popliteal veins in her left leg. Computed tomography (CT) of the abdominal and pelvis showed a mass in the pelvis, periaortic lymphadenopathy, and several lesions in the liver compatible with metastases. A colonoscopy with biopsy confirms recurrent adenocarcinoma of the colon.

Anticoagulant therapy is contraindicated in patients with active, potentially life-threatening bleeding. Without anticoagulant therapy, extension of the thrombus will likely occur, especially in cancer patients with active malignancy. Many clinicians recommend insertion of an IVC filter in this setting. However, this approach does not suppress the thrombotic process or relieve the symptoms of VTE, and fatal PE has been reported. If a filter is being considered, patients should be made aware of the potential for no benefit or worsening of symptoms. In the end-of-life setting, insertion of a filter should be avoided as clear benefits to the patient are yet to be demonstrated.

In patients with mild bleeding from sources that are not potentially life threatening, the use of LMWH may be considered for relieving symptoms of VTE. The patient should be hospitalized, started on a prophylactic dose of a LMWH, and monitored for any increase in bleeding. If bleeding does not worsen, the dose can be increased slowly with an aim to control VTE symptoms. The dose is kept at the lowest level that provides symptomatic relief. If bleeding increases, LMWH should be held for a few days. When the bleeding reduces and is stable again, a lower dose of LMWH can be restarted. This trial and error approach requires patience and thorough education and cooperation of the patient. Alternatively, some clinicians prefer using intravenous heparin in this setting because of its rapid reversibility if bleeding worsens. The difficulty with this approach is changing over to long-term treatment.

In this patient, LMWH therapy is a reasonable first option. Because her DVT symptoms are minimal, subtherapeutic doses of LMWH may reduce symptoms, and suppress extension of the thrombus, without exacerbating her bleeding. Insertion of a filter may worsen her symptoms and should be avoided. It is also important to obtain advice from oncology and gynecology services to stop the bleeding from her vaginal lesion.

Case 2: patient with severe thrombocytopenia and need for anticoagulation

A 55-year-old man with non-small-cell lung cancer presents with shortness of breath and pleuritic chest pain. He is receiving experimental chemotherapy and has required red cell transfusion support because of severe marrow suppression. His platelet count has also been low, fluctuating between 30–50×10^9/L but he has had no bleeding episodes.

Significant findings on physical examination include a sinus tachycardia of 110 beats per minute, an oxygen saturation of 96 per cent on room air, a fever of 37.9°C, and absent breath sounds at the left base. A chest X-ray is consistent with an effusion and consolidation of the left lower lobe. A CT pulmonary angiogram shows bilateral PE with infarction of his left lower lobe and a moderate-size pleural effusion. His legs have no symptoms of DVT and a compression ultrasound did not show evidence of DVT. His blood count shows a leukocyte count of 2.1×10^9/L, hemoglobin of 85 g/L and his platelet count is 33×10^9/L.

Anticoagulation is indicated in this patient because of the extent of his acute PE. He is hemodynamically stable and does not warrant thrombolysis. His low grade fever is likely secondary to his pulmonary infarction, although infection as the source cannot be absolutely ruled out. Because of his thrombocytopenia, extra caution must be applied when anticoagulants are used. It is not documented in the literature whether full dose anticoagulation is well tolerated in patients with thrombocytopenia, and whether there is a cut-off value below which anticoagulants are contraindicated.

Anecdotally, therapeutic doses of LMWH have been used in patients with platelet counts above 50×10^9/L without an increased incidence of serious bleeding. Because bleeding in a patient on therapeutic doses of anticoagulants occurs only if there is a source of bleeding, it is possible that anticoagulation is tolerated at even lower platelet count values. However, below a count of 20×10^9/L, most clinicians would be hesitant to recommend anticoagulation.

In this patient, it is reasonable to transfuse the patient with platelets to maintain the platelet count above 50×10^9/L and proceed with full dose anticoagulation with LMWH. Unless the patient is refractory to platelet transfusions, this supportive effort will often allow full dose anticoagulation for the first month, when the risk of thrombus extension or recurrent PE is highest. Once this period is over, then a reduced dose of LMWH is administered and it might be possible to allow the platelet count to stay above 20×10^9/L. If it is not possible to maintain the platelet count above 20×10^9/L, with or without transfusions, continuing therapy with a prophylactic dose of LMWH is an option. Such a low dose has been used successfully for prophylaxis for veno-occlusive disease in patients undergoing allogeneic bone marrow transplantation.

Case 3: patient with recurrent PE while receiving LMWH

A 72-year-old man with metastatic cholangiocarcinoma presents with increasing shortness of breath and right leg swelling. He was diagnosed with an acute DVT of his right leg 2 months ago based on a positive ultrasound. He was given dalteparin at 200 IU per kg once daily for the first month followed by dalteparin at 150 IU per kg once daily. He has been compliant with his injections and has had no problems with bleeding or bruising. He noted marked improvement in his leg symptoms after starting on dalteparin.

After reducing his dose of dalteparin, however, the patient has noticed increasing swelling of his leg. Two days ago, he noticed marked shortness of breath with minimal exertion. He was not able to walk up a flight of stairs without having to stop half way to catch his breath. Today, he is having difficulty breathing while sitting down and watching television. He presented promptly to the emergency department.

Upon arrival at the emergency department, his vital signs were unremarkable except for sinus tachycardia at 120 beats per minute. His oxygen saturation was 92 per cent on room air. His lung examination showed no wheezing or crackles. His right leg was swollen. He underwent a number of tests, including an ECG, chest X-ray, a CT pulmonary angiogram, and ultrasonography of his legs. Extension of his DVT was confirmed and bilateral filling defects were seen in lobar and segmental pulmonary arteries in both lungs, indicating acute PE.

Based on the CLOT study and other prospective studies, approximately 9 per cent of patients with cancer and VTE treated with LMWH will develop symptomatic recurrence or extension of their thrombus. The most appropriate treatment for these patients is not known. The options include increasing the dose of LMWH, switching to UFH, or inserting an IVC filter. The most convenient and logical approach is to increase the dose of LMWH. As discussed earlier, using an IVC filter is not appropriate.

In patients who develop recurrence while receiving a subtherapeutic dose of LMWH, the dose should be raised back to weight-based therapeutic levels. This is often sufficient to provide symptomatic relief and prevent further thrombus extension.

In patients who develop recurrence while receiving a therapeutic dose of LMWH, then an empiric dose increase of 25 per cent is reasonable. Re-assessment should be done in 5 to 7 days. If the symptoms improve, then the patient remains on the higher dose of LMWH. If the symptoms have not improved, then the dose should be increased again. At this point, it is useful to look at the anti-factor Xa level at 3 hours after an injection to help guide further dose increases. If the anti-Xa level is low, then a substantial increase in the LMWH dose can be tolerated. If the level is near the upper limit of the therapeutic range, then smaller increments of LMWH is prudent. It has been shown that some patients require higher than the usual recommended weight-based doses of LMWH to achieve conventional therapeutic anti-Xa levels. The reason for this is unknown but it may be related to a greater degree of nonspecific binding of LMWH in patients with aggressive disease, in whom plasma levels of acute phase reactants would likely be very elevated.

In this patient, administration of the full therapeutic dose of LMWH is the appropriate course of action. Reduction of his LMWH dose in the future is not recommended as the risk of recurrence VTE will be high.

Case 4: patient admitted for end-of-life care with increasing leg swelling

A 41-year-old woman is admitted to the hospital for pain control and end-of-life care. She has advanced gastroesophageal carcinoma that was diagnosed approximately 3 months ago, after several months of progressive dysphagia and odynophagia. Staging investigations showed that she had extensive unresectable disease. She refused standard chemotherapy and radiation but received alternative medicine from an herbalist. She has lost about 40 lbs in the past 6 months. She also has had melena in the past but there has been no recent episodes noted.

About a week ago her husband noticed swelling around her left ankle but the patient denies having pain or discomfort in the leg. She has had no difficulties with her breathing but she admits to being short of breath on exertion. She denies any chest pain, hemoptysis, fever, or chills. Her only complaint is pain in her back. Her leg swelling is not bothersome and her activity level is very limited. She is receiving morphine and gabapentin. Her husband has been caring for her and their three young children. He is having difficulty coping at home but he wants to respect her wish to die at home.

On examination, the patient appears to be comfortable. Vital signs are within normal limits. The most obvious abnormality is her left leg, which was very swollen compared to the right. The left leg is slightly dusky. There is significant pitting edema in the left leg. Her left calf is firm but non-tender to palpation.

A compression B-mode ultrasound confirms the presence of occlusive thrombus extending from the left external iliac vein, the common femoral vein, all the way down to the trifurcation of the calf.

Extensive thrombosis can sometimes be relatively asymptomatic. In the end-of-life setting where palliation of symptoms is the primary goal, it is reasonable to not administer anticoagulant therapy if the treatment was felt to be burdensome or reduce the quality of life. Daily injection with a LMWH is relatively straight forward but can exacerbate bleeding. Administration of warfarin with laboratory monitoring should be avoided. Insertion of an IVC filter has no role. Frank and thorough discussions with the family and patient are needed to understand their needs and formulate a care plan that would be acceptable to all. Withholding anticoagulation and judicious use of analgesics may be the optimal approach in some cases.

References

1. Levitan N, Dowlati A, Remick SC *et al.* Rates of initial and recurrent thromboembolic disease among patients with malignancy versus those without malignancy. Risk analysis using Medicare claims data. *Medicine (Baltimore)* 1999;78(5):285–91.

2. Sorensen HT, Mellemkjaer L, Olsen JH *et al.* Prognosis of cancers associated with venous thromboembolism. *The New England Journal of Medicine* 2000;343(25):1846–50.

3. Altinbas M, Coskun HS, Er O *et al.* A randomized clinical trial of combination chemotherapy with and without low-molecular-weight heparin in small cell lung cancer. *Journal of Thrombosis and Haemostasis* 2004;2(8):1266–71.

4. Kakkar AK, Levine MN, Kadziola Z *et al.* Low molecular weight heparin therapy with dalteparin and survival in advanced cancer: the Fragmin Advanced Malignancy Outcome Study (FAMOUS). *Journal of Clinical Oncology* 2004;22(10):1944–8.

5. Klerk CP, Smorenburg SM, Otten HM *et al.* The effect of low molecular weight heparin on survival in patients with advanced malignancy. *Journal of Clinical Oncology* 2005;23(10):2130–5.

6. Lee AY, Rickles FR, Julian JA *et al.* Randomized comparison of low molecular weight heparin and coumarin derivatives on the survival of patients with cancer and venous thromboembolism. *Journal of Clinical Oncology* 2005;23(10):2123–9.

7. Buller HR, Davidson BL, Decousus H *et al.* Subcutaneous fondaparinux versus intravenous unfractionated heparin in the initial treatment of pulmonary embolism. *The New England Journal of Medicine* 2003;349(18):1695–702.

8. Buller HR, Davidson BL, Decousus H *et al.* Fondaparinux or enoxaparin for the initial treatment of symptomatic deep venous thrombosis: a randomized trial. *Annals of Internal Medicine* 2004;140(11):867–73.

9. The van Gogh Investigators. Idraparinux versus standard therapy for venous thromboembolic disease. *The New England Journal of Medicine* 2007;357:1094–104.

10. The van Gogh Investigators. Extended prophylaxis of venous thromboembolism with idraparinux. *The New England Journal of Medicine* 2007;357:1105–12.

11. van Dongen CJ, van den Belt AG, Prins MH *et al.* Fixed dose subcutaneous low molecular weight heparins versus adjusted dose unfractionated heparin for venous thromboembolism. *Cochrane Database of Systematic Reviews* 2004;(4):CD001100.

12. Buller HR, Agnelli G, Hull RD *et al.* Antithrombotic therapy for venous thromboembolic disease: the Seventh ACCP Conference on Antithrombotic and Thrombolytic Therapy. *Chest* 2004;126(3 Suppl):401S–28S.

13. Kearon C, Ginsberg JS, Julian JA *et al.* Comparison of fixed-dose weight-adjusted unfractionated heparin and low-molecular-weight heparin for acute treatment of venous thromboembolism. *The Journal of the American Medical Association* 2006;296(8):935–42.

14. Levine M, Gent M, Hirsh J *et al.* A comparison of low-molecular-weight heparin administered primarily at home with unfractionated heparin administered in the hospital for proximal deep-vein thrombosis. *The New England Journal of Medicine* 1996;334(11):677–81.

15. Koopman MM, Prandoni P, Piovella F *et al.* Treatment of venous thrombosis with intravenous unfractionated heparin administered in the hospital as compared with subcutaneous low- molecular-weight heparin administered at home. The Tasman Study Group [published erratum appears in The New England Journal of Medicine 1997 Oct 23;337(17):1251]. *The New England Journal of Medicine* 1996;334(11):682–7.

16. Columbus Investigators. Low-molecular-weight heparin in the treatment of patients with venous thromboembolism. The Columbus Investigators. *The New England Journal of Medicine* 1997;337(10):657–62.

17. Merli G, Spiro TE, Olsson CG *et al.* Subcutaneous enoxaparin once or twice daily compared with intravenous unfractionated heparin for treatment of venous thromboembolic disease. *Annals of Internal Medicine* 2001;134(3):191–202.

18. Wells PS, Kovacs MJ, Bormanis J *et al.* Expanding eligibility for outpatient treatment of deep venous thrombosis and pulmonary embolism with low-molecular-weight heparin: a comparison of patient self-injection with homecare injection. *Archives of Internal Medicine* 1998;158(16):1809–12.

19. Harrison L, McGinnis J, Crowther M *et al.* Assessment of outpatient treatment of deep-vein thrombosis with low- molecular-weight heparin. *Archives of Internal Medicine* 1998;158(18):2001–3.

20. O'Shaughnessy D, Miles J, Wimperis J. UK patients with deep-vein thrombosis can be safely treated as out-patients. *The Quarterly Journal of Medicine* 2000;93(10):663–7.

21. Ageno W, Steidl L, Marchesi C *et al.* Selecting patients for home treatment of deep vein thrombosis: the problem of cancer. *Haematologica* 2002;87(3):286–91.

22. Avritscher EB, Cantor SB, Shih YC *et al.* Cost-minimization analysis of low-molecular-weight heparin (dalteparin) compared to unfractionated heparin for inpatient treatment of cancer patients with deep venous thrombosis. *Supportive Care in Cancer* 2004;12(7):531–6.

23. Breddin HK, Hach-Wunderle V, Nakov R *et al.* Effects of a low-molecular-weight heparin on thrombus regression and recurrent thromboembolism in patients with deep-vein thrombosis. *The New England Journal of Medicine* 2001;344(9):626–31.

24. Prandoni P, Lensing AW, Piccioli A *et al.* Recurrent venous thromboembolism and bleeding complications during anticoagulant treatment in patients with cancer and venous thrombosis. *Blood* 2002;100(10):3484–8.

25. Hutten BA, Prins MH, Gent M *et al.* Incidence of recurrent thromboembolic and bleeding complications among patients with venous thromboembolism in relation to both malignancy and achieved international normalized ratio: a retrospective analysis. *Journal of Clinical Oncology* 2000;18(17):3078–83.

26. Gates S, Brocklehurst P, Davis LJ. Prophylaxis for venous thromboembolic disease in pregnancy and the early postnatal period. *Cochrane Database of Systematic Reviews* 2002;(2):CD001689.

27. Rodger MA, Kahn SR, Cranney A *et al.* Long-term dalteparin in pregnancy not associated with a decrease in bone mineral density: substudy of a randomized controlled trial. *Journal of Thrombosis and Haemostasis* 2007;5(8):1600–6.

28. Meyer G, Marjanovic Z, Valcke J *et al.* Comparison of low-molecular-weight heparin and warfarin for the secondary prevention of venous thromboembolism in patients with cancer: a randomized controlled study. *Archives of Internal Medicine* 2002;162(15):1729–35.

29. Deitcher SR, Kessler CM, Merli G *et al.* Secondary prevention of venous thromboembolic events in patients with active cancer: enoxaparin alone versus initial enoxaparin followed by warfarin for a 180-day period. *Clinical and Applied Thrombosis/Haemostasis* 2006;12(4):389–96.

30. Lee AY, Levine MN, Baker RI *et al.* Low-molecular-weight heparin versus a coumarin for the prevention of recurrent venous thromboembolism in patients with cancer. *The New England Journal of Medicine* 2003;349(2):146–53.

31. Monreal M, Zacharski L, Jimenez JA *et al.* Fixed-dose low-molecular-weight heparin for secondary prevention of venous thromboembolism in patients with disseminated cancer: a prospective cohort study. *Journal of Thrombosis and Haemostasis* 2004;2(8):1311–15.

32. Hull RD, Pineo GF, Brant RF *et al.* Long-term low-molecular-weight heparin versus usual care in proximal-vein thrombosis patients with cancer. *The American Journal of Medicine* 2006;119(12):1062–72.

33. Baglin TP, Keeling DM, Watson HG. Guidelines on oral anticoagulation (warfarin): third edition—2005 update. *British Journal of Haematology* 2006;132(3):277–85.

34. Mandala M, Falanga A, Piccioli A *et al.* Venous thromboembolism and cancer: guidelines of the Italian Association of Medical Oncology (AIOM). *Critical Reviews in Oncology/Hematology* 2006;59(3):194–204.

35. Wagman LD, Baird MF, Bennett CL *et al.* Venous thromboembolic disease. Clinical practice guidelines in oncology. *Journal of the National Comprehensive Cancer Network* 2006;4(9):838–69.

36. Lyman GH, Khorana AA, Falanga A *et al.* American Society of Clinical Oncology guideline: recommendations for venous thromboembolism prophylaxis and treatment in patients with cancer. *Journal of Clinical Oncology* 2007;25(34):5490–505.

37. Noble SIR, Hood K, Finlay IG. The use of long-term low-molecular-weight heparin for the treatment of venous thromboembolism in palliative care patets with advanced cancer: a case series of 62 patients. *Palliative Medicine* 2007;21(6):473–6.

38. Chan A, Woodruff RK. Complications and failure of anticoagulation therapy in the treatment of venous thromboembolism in patients with disseminated malignancy. *Australian and New Zealand Journal of Medicine* 1992;22(2):119–22.

39. Harrington KJ, Bateman AR, Syrigos KN *et al.* Cancer-related thromboembolic disease in patients with solid tumours: a retrospective analysis. *Annals of Oncology* 1997;8(7):669–73.

40. Luk C, Wells PS, Anderson D *et al.* Extended outpatient therapy with low molecular weight heparin for the treatment of recurrent venous thromboembolism despite warfarin therapy. *The American Journal of Medicine* 2001;111(4):270–3.

41. Decousus H, Leizorovicz A, Parent F *et al.* A clinical trial of vena caval filters in the prevention of pulmonary embolism in patients with proximal deep-vein thrombosis. Prevention du Risque d'Embolie Pulmonaire par Interruption Cave Study Group. *The New England Journal of Medicine* 1998;338(7):409–15.

42. PREPIC Investigators. Eight-year follow-up of patients with permanent vena cava filters in the prevention of pulmonary embolism: the PREPIC (Prevention du Risque d'Embolie Pulmonaire par Interruption Cave) randomized study. *Circulation* 2005;112(3):416–22.

43. White RH, Zhou H, Kim J *et al.* A population-based study of the effectiveness of inferior vena cava filter use among patients with venous thromboembolism. *Archives of Internal Medicine* 2000;160(13):2033–41.

44. Streiff MB. Vena caval filters: a comprehensive review. Blood 2000;95(12):3669–77.

45. Getzen TM, Rectenwald JE. Inferior vena cava filters in the cancer patient: current use and indications. *Journal of the National Comprehensive Cancer Network* 2006;4(9):881–8.

46. Elting LS, Escalante CP, Cooksley C *et al.* Outcomes and cost of deep venous thrombosis among patients with cancer. *Archives of Internal Medicine* 2004;164(15):1653–61.

47. Wallace MJ, Jean JL, Gupta S *et al.* Use of inferior vena caval filters and survival in patients with malignancy. *Cancer* 2004;101(8):1902–7.

48. Schunn C, Schunn GB, Hobbs G *et al.* Inferior vena cava filter placement in late-stage cancer. *Vascular and Endovascular Surgery* 2006;40(4):287–94.

49. Jarrett BP, Dougherty MJ, Calligaro KD. Inferior vena cava filters in malignant disease. *Journal of Vascular Surgery* 2002;36(4):704–7.

50. Rickles FR, Shoji M, Abe K. The role of the hemostatic system in tumor growth, metastasis, and angiogenesis: tissue factor is a bifunctional molecule capable of inducing both fibrin deposition and angiogenesis in cancer. *International Journal of Hematology* 2001;73(2):145–50.

51. Noble SIR, Finlay IG. Is long-term low-molecular-weight heparin acceptable to palliative care patients in the treatment of cancer related venous thromboembolism? A qualitative study. *Palliative Medicine* 2005;19(3):197–201.

52. Hull RD, Pineo GF, Mah AF *et al.* Long-term out-of-hospital treatment with low-molecular-weight heparin versus warfarin sodium: a randomized trial comparing the quality of life associated with these antithrombotic therapies. *Blood* 2001;98(11):267a.

53. Hull RD, Pineo GF, Mah AF *et al.* A randomized trial evaluating long-term low-molecular-weight heparin therapy out-of-hospital versus warfarin sodium comparing the post-phlebitic outcomes at three months. *Blood* 2001;98:447a

Chapter 7

Primary thromboprophylaxis in the advanced cancer patient

Simon I.R. Noble

Introduction

Prevention or primary prophylaxis of venous thromboembolism (VTE) in palliative care remains a contentious issue. The heterogeneity of the palliative-care population makes it inappropriate to adopt a 'one size fits all' policy. No adequately powered and recruited clinical trials have been conducted in a representative population and the outcome measures used in other clinical studies may not be wholly appropriate in the palliative setting. In addition, the aim of thromboprophylaxis in most settings is to provide temporary anticoagulation until a risk of VTE is over. However, in case of patients with advanced and progressive cancer, the risk will be ongoing and it is difficult to know when it would be beneficial to initiate thromboprophylaxis for an increased risk over and above this baseline risk, and when to stop it. The lack of consensus is reflected by an absence of clinical guidelines within palliative care and a variation of thromboprophylaxis practice amongst specialist palliative-care units (SPCUs).[1] Chapter 2 has already outlined the breadth of histology, performance status, metastatic spread, and coexistent pathology that defines the palliative-care cancer population. In addition to physical status, patients will have differing spiritual and psychosocial needs that will influence their treatment goals and thus the clinical decision-making process. This chapter will review the current published evidence available that may guide the clinician in the appropriate use of primary thromboprophylaxis and, where possible, apply this evidence to care in the advanced cancer patient.

This chapter recognizes that patients cared for in SPCUs across the world will vary. Some palliative-care services will look after patients throughout their cancer journey, whilst other units may focus solely on end-of-life care. Regardless of where a palliative inpatient receives their care—in an acute hospital, hospice, or community—their thrombotic risk will be similar. Management should not be based on blanket policy but a measured individualized team decision, and where appropriate, in conjunction with the patient themselves.

In this chapter, the main studies that guide clinical practice in surgery and medicine shall be reviewed and their applicability to the palliative-care setting discussed. Following this, suggestions for the prevention of VTE in the real world palliative-care setting shall be considered, followed by discussion of some clinical cases.

Current practice in the general medical and surgical population

Prophylaxis of VTE in general medical and surgical patients should, in theory, be straightforward since it is guided by several well-conducted randomized controlled trials (RCTs) with outcome measures appropriate to their respective populations.[2] However, the thromboprophylaxis of hospitalized patients varies worldwide. The ENDORSE investigators recently assessed admissions to 358 hospitals across 32 countries for risk and subsequent prophylaxis of VTE according to 2004 American College of Chest Physicians (ACCP) evidence-based consensus guidelines.[3] Out of 68,183 patients, 30,827 (45 per cent) were surgical, 37,356 (55 per cent) were medical, and 35,329 (51.8 per cent) were judged to be at risk for VTE. This comprised 19,842 (64.4 per cent) surgical and 15,487 (41.5 per cent) medical patients. Of the surgical patients at risk, 11,613 (58.5 per cent) received VTE prophylaxis, compared with 6,119 (39.5 per cent) at-risk medical patients. An ongoing multinational prospective observational study of 15,156 by the IMPROVE investigators suggests only 60 per cent of patients, who either meet the ACCP criteria for prophylaxis or are eligible for enrolment in randomized clinical trials that have shown the benefits of pharmacologic prophylaxis, actually receive prophylaxis.[4]

The presence of cancer is recognized as an independent risk factor for VTE[5,6] and the National Comprehensive Cancer Network (NCCN) guidelines,[7] Seventh ACCP guidelines,[8] and the latest International Union of Angioplasty (IUA) guidelines,[9] all categorize hospitalized cancer patients as a group at high or highest risk for VTE who should receive pharmacological thromboprophylaxis, unless contraindicated. Despite this, thromboprophylaxis in cancer patients varies worldwide and there is an underappreciation, even amongst some oncologists, of the thrombotic risks of the malignant state.[10] A 4-year retrospective study across the US revealed low rates of thromboprophylaxis for medically ill patients, including those with cancer, who were at high risk for VTE.[11] The use of prophylaxis in cancer patients improved slightly between 2001 and 2004, from 18 to 25 per cent, but still remained at an unacceptably low percentage. The Fundamental Research in Oncology and Thrombosis (FRONTLINE) survey, which assessed worldwide opinions and prescribing practices relating to VTE in cancer patients, suggested routine thromboprophylaxis occurs in over 50 per cent of surgical oncology patients, but in less than 5 per cent of medical oncology inpatients.[12] A recent Canadian multicenter hospital audit of thromboprophylaxis use in medical inpatients found that patients admitted for cancer were significantly less likely to receive any form of VTE prophylaxis than other medical patients (OR, 0.40; 95 per cent CI, 0.24–0.68; $P = 0.0007$).[13]

Evidence in specific populations

General cancer surgery

The majority of evidence in cancer thromboprophylaxis is from surgical studies. The role of surgical procedures, such as palliative stoma formation, is increasing. Likewise, many palliative-care services are involved in the care of surgical oncology patients earlier in their cancer journey, for symptom control and rehabilitation. The risk of VTE in patients undergoing surgery for cancer may be as high as 50 per cent without prophylaxis.[14] Anticoagulant prophylaxis is routinely recommended for patients undergoing major surgery as a single preoperative injection of a heparin (unfractionated heparin [UFH] or a low molecular weight heparin [LMWH]), followed by subcutaneous injections starting within 12–24 h after surgery. UFH is given two or three times daily while LMWH requires only once-a-day injections. It is important to consider the impact such differences may have in terms of in terms of patient comfort, nursing time, and the likelihood of potential drug error. In patients who have a high risk of bleeding, prophylaxis with compression stockings is often used as alternative, but it is less effective than anticoagulant prophylaxis, especially in high-risk patients.[14,15] Prophylaxis is continued usually for few days during the patients' stay in hospital. A meta-analysis published by Mismetti and colleagues suggests once-daily LMWH to be as efficacious and safe as multidose UFH in patients with cancer undergoing major surgery.[16] This included data from the ENOXACAN study that compared LMWH with UFH in 631 evaluable patients undergoing elective, curative surgery for colorectal cancer.[17] Enoxaparin 40 mg, injected once a day and UFH 5,000 U, given three times a day, were started 2 h before surgery. No difference was detected between the two groups for the primary endpoint venographically detected deep vein thrombosis (DVT) and symptomatic VTE at the end of the tenth-day treatment period (14.7 vs. 18.2 per cent, respectively). Major bleeding was reported in 3–4 per cent in both patient groups and a difference in mortality was not observed.

The ENOXACAN II trial examined the efficacy and safety of extended prophylaxis with LMWH beyond hospitalization in cancer patients.[18] In this multicentre, double-blind, placebo-controlled trial, 501 patients undergoing elective, curative abdominal, or pelvic surgery for cancer were randomized and 332 were evaluable for the primary outcome. All patients received enoxaparin 40 mg once daily for the first 6–10 days after surgery, the first dose given 10–14 h before surgery. After the initial postoperative period on enoxaparin, patients were then randomized to continue with enoxaparin 40 mg once daily or placebo injections until bilateral venography was performed between 25 and 31 days after surgery. The primary outcome was DVT detected on bilateral venography and symptomatic VTE. During the treatment period, 12.0 per cent (20 of 167) of the placebo patients compared with 4.8 per cent (8 of 165) of the enoxaparin patients had a confirmed thrombotic event ($P = 0.02$). One patient had confirmed pulmonary embolism (PE). Extended prophylaxis with enoxaparin significantly reduced the rate of VTE by 60 per cent (95 per cent CI, 10–82 per cent). During the double-blinded period, major bleeding occurred in none of the patients in the placebo group and 0.4 per cent in the enoxaparin group.

More recently fondaparinux has been evaluated in patients undergoing high-risk abdominal surgery.[19] In the PEGASUS trial, a phase III, double-blind, double-dummy trial, 2,927 patients undergoing major abdominal surgery were randomized to receive once-daily injections of fondaparinux 2.5 mg or dalteparin 5,000 U. There was no difference in the incidence of VTE in both groups although in a *post hoc* analysis of the subgroup of 1,408 patients with cancer, fondaparinux was associated with a statistically significant reduction in VTE compared with dalteparin (4.7 vs. 7.7 per cent; $P = 0.02$).

Gynaecological surgery

Prophylaxis in women undergoing surgery for gynaecological malignancies has been studied in small cohort studies and randomized trials.[20–26] A Cochrane database meta-analysis of the pharmacological thromboprophylaxis agents found that UFH and LMWH are both effective in preventing DVT compared with placebo (OR 0.30, 95 per cent CI, 0.10–0.89) and that they appear to be equally effective.[27] However, there is no evidence as yet to suggest that heparin, warfarin, or aspirin reduce the incidence of PE.

Neurosurgery

Neurosurgery for central nervous system malignancies has a risk of thrombosis up to 60 per cent in the immediate postoperative period.[28,29] Two random-ized trials have shown that LMWH prophylaxis started after neurosurgery can reduce the risk of VTE without increasing serious bleeding. About 80 per cent of the patients in these trials were undergoing neurosurgery for malignancy. In one trial, patients were randomized to nadroparin or placebo starting at 18–24 h after surgery.[30] Mandatory bilateral venography detected DVT in 31 of 166 patients (18.7 per cent) assigned to nadroparin compared with 47 of 179 patients (26.3 per cent) randomized to placebo ($P = 0.047$). Major bleeding was reported in six and two patients respectively ($P = 0.087$). Mortality was significantly higher in the nadroparin group, but none of the deaths were judged to be related to drug study. In another placebo-controlled randomized trial, comparing enoxaparin 40 mg once daily starting within 24 h after surgery compared with placebo demonstrated a reduction in VTE risk by 47 per cent; 22 of 153 patients (17 per cent) vs. 42 of 154 patients (32 per cent), respectively.[31] In this trial, no differences in bleeding and overall mortality were observed and in both studies, all patients also wore graduated compression stockings. A meta-analysis, which included these trials, reported that prophylaxis with LMWH resulted in a 38 per cent relative risk reduction of VTE ($P < 0.001$) without an excessive increase in the bleeding risk.(32)

Spinal cord injury

Acute spinal cord compression (SCC) occurs in 5 per cent of cancer patients, many of whom are of good performance status prior to presentation.[33] Of those treated with radiotherapy or surgery, over 68 per cent will be discharged from hospital of which 78 per cent will go home.[33] Whilst the presentation of cord compression represents progression of malignant disease, the 3- and 6-month survival outcomes are 35 and 20 per cent, respectively. Without prophylaxis, patients with acute SCC have a very high risk of developing VTE since they have an acute spinal cord injury (SCI), malignancy, and are immobile. Asymptomatic DVT occurs in 60–100 per cent of SCI patients who are subject to routine screening.[35–37] Small randomized trials suggest low dose UFH (LDUH) or intermittent pneumatic compression (IPC) is ineffective in VTE prophylaxis while adjusted-dose UFH and LMWH are substantially more efficacious.[2]

In a large multicentre study of 476 patients with acute SCI enrolled in 27 centres, patients were randomized to receive either the combination of UFH 5,000 units tds plus IPC (LDUH-IPC) or enoxaparin 30 mg bd.[38] DVT was demonstrated in 63 per cent of the LDUH-IPC group and in 66 per cent of the enoxaparin patients. The rates of major VTE (either proximal DVT or PE) were 16 and 12 per cent, respectively, although no patient died of PE. Major bleeding was seen in 5 per cent of LDUH-IPC patients and in 3 per cent of those who received enoxaparin.

Medical inpatients

Although VTE is most often considered to be associated with recent surgery or trauma, 50–70 per cent of symptomatic thromboembolic events and

70–80 per cent of fatal PEs occur in nonsurgical patients.[2] Hospitalization for an acute medical illness is independently associated with about an 8-fold increased relative risk for VTE, and accounts for almost one-quarter of all VTE events within the general population.[39]

There is less data on the safety and efficacy of thromboprophylaxis in hospitalized medical cancer patients. However, clinical trials in hospitalized general medical patients (Table 7.1), which included cancer patients demonstrate that LMWH prophylaxis leads to a lower VTE incidence compared with placebo, without increasing major bleeding.[40,41] A meta-analysis of randomized trials comparing LMWHs and UFH in medical inpatients reported that the two regimens were similarly effective in reducing VTE events. In this analysis, the incidence of major haemorrhage was 52 per cent lower in patients who received prophylactic LMWH compared with low-dose UFH ($P = 0.049$).[42]

The thromboprophylaxis efficacy of the synthetic factor Xa inhibitor fondaparinux, 2.5 mg subcutaneously once daily, was assessed in a blinded, placebo-controlled study in 849 acutely ill medical patients, 14 per cent of whom had cancer.[43] The primary outcome, a combination of DVT detected by routine venogram and symptomatic VTE, occurred in 10.5 and 5.6 per cent, respectively, of the patients who received placebo and fondaparinux ($P < 0.029$). Fatal PE was also significantly reduced in the fondaparinux recipients (5 vs. 0 events). Major bleeding was seen in 0.2 per cent of patients in both groups.

Oncology outpatients receiving palliative chemotherapy

Advancements in anticancer therapies have improved the long-term prognosis of many patients with advanced malignancy. Patients with metastatic disease from sites such as breast, prostate, and colorectal cancer, are living longer and the palliative stages of some cancers share similarities with chronic diseases. Although there are few data on the thromboprophylaxis of ambulant cancer patients, some specific cancer patients have been studied.

In a placebo-controlled study, women with stage IV breast cancer were randomized to receive low-dose warfarin or placebo for the duration of their multiagent chemotherapy.[44] Warfarin was given at 1 mg daily for 6 weeks

Table 7.1 LMWH thromboprophylaxis studies in acutely hospitalized medical patients.

Study name	Number in study (N)	N with cancer (per cent)	Placebo events (per cent)	Treatment events (per cent)	Relative risk	P	95 per cent CI
MEDENOX[40]	579	12.4	14.9	5.5	0.37	<0.001	0.22–0.63
PREVENT[41]	3,706	5.1	4.96	2.77	0.55	0.0015	0.38–0.8

and then the dose was adjusted to maintain the international normalized ratio (INR) at 1.3–1.9. Seven of 159 patients receiving placebo compared with one of 152 taking warfarin, developed symptomatic, objectively confirmed thromboembolic events. The relative risk reduction of 85 per cent associated with warfarin use was statistically significant ($P = 0.03$). No difference in any or major bleeding was found, with a total of five patients in the placebo group and eight patients in the warfarin group having had any bleeding. Whilst these results are impressive, this regimen of prophylaxis is rarely used. Several reasons have been suggested including a poor tolerability of patients to repeated INR monitoring. It has also been suggested that the relatively low risk of VTE in the control group calls into question whether routine prophylaxis is warranted, especially as it confers a bleeding risk equal to the risk of VTE.

Myeloma patients receiving thalidomide or lenalidomide, especially in combination with dexamethasone or chemotherapy are at particular risk of developing VTE.[45] There are data to support the use of LMWH, full-dose warfarin, and aspirin as primary prophylactic agents, but no studies have been conducted comparing the agents.[46]

Application of the evidence to palliative-care patients

There is very little data on primary prophylaxis in the palliative-care literature, and its benefit in the SPCU setting is yet to be demonstrated. Thromboprophylaxis with LMWH appears to be an acceptable intervention to patients with advanced malignancy, yet health care professionals may consider routine thromboprophylaxis culturally challenging.[47,48] In order to understand the case for thromboprophylaxis—if indeed there is one—in the palliative-care setting, one must first understand the reasons for thromboprophylaxis in the general population. Table 7.2 outlines the rationale for thromboprophylaxis on the grounds that VTE is common yet easily preventable. Prophylaxis is cost-effective and prevents fatal as well as symptomatic thrombotic events. However, in the palliative-care setting, where the intention is 'neither to hasten or postpone death',[49] the decision to initiate an intervention with the sole aim of preventing death in a terminally ill patient may be viewed as countercultural to the philosophy of the speciality. The corollary to this lies with the appreciation that as palliative care has developed as a specialty, patients are being looked after by palliative-care services earlier in their disease journey, and not all SPCU admissions are for terminal care. Many will be admitted for management of complex symptoms with the intention of discharging them back to their usual place of care. Admissions may be precipitated by acute events such as hypercalcaemia, SCC, heart failure, or pneumonia, which as well as being reversible pathologies, are also prothrombotic and worthy of

Table 7.2 Rationale for thromboprophylaxis in general population.

High prevalence of VTE:

♦ Most hospitalized patients have risk factors for VTE

♦ DVT is common in many hospitalized patient groups

Adverse consequences of unprevented VTE:

♦ Symptomatic DVT and PE

♦ Fatal PE

♦ Cost of investigating symptomatic patients

♦ Risk of treated unprevented VTE, that is, bleeding

♦ Post-thrombotic syndrome

Efficacy and effectiveness of thromboprophylaxis:

♦ Thromboprophylaxis is highly efficacious at preventing DVT and proximal DVT

♦ Thromboprophylaxis is highly effective at preventing symptomatic VTE and fatal PE

♦ Cost-effectiveness of prophylaxis has repeatedly been demonstrated

prophylaxis in a general medical setting. It could be argued that patients with reversible pathology should be considered for thromboprophylaxis—especially since there is evidence to support this—in the general population and the thrombotic risk increases with disease progression.[50]

Another barrier to thromboprophylaxis lies with a belief that it is less of a problem in the palliative-care setting than the literature may suggest.[51] The estimated perceived incidence of VTE in the palliative-care setting has been reported at 1–5 per cent, which is likely to be an underestimate.[52] A prospective study of 258 hospice inpatients, assessed using light reflection rheography suggested a prevalence of VTE in 52 per cent of patients (95 per cent CI, 46–58) and 9 per cent of the total sample had objectively confirmed symptomatic VTE.[53] Of those diagnosed with asymptomatic DVT 32 per cent went on to develop symptoms consistent with DVT ($P<0.001$) and 13 per cent symptoms suggestive of PE ($P<0.02$) over a median of 36-day follow-up.[54] It is likely that symptomatic VTE is being underdiagnosed in the advanced cancer patient, which is unsurprising since the symptoms of DVT and PE mimic those of other pathological processes, which may be considered before a diagnosis of VTE (Tables 7.3 and 7.4). Whether undiagnosed VTE is being labelled as asymptomatic since other processes could account for such symptoms is yet to be evaluated. It could be argued that thromboprophylaxis is appropriate in selected patients if only to prevent distressing symptoms such as dyspnoea. It is difficult to identify which patients would benefit from being selected since almost all palliative-care patients would qualify for

Table 7.3 Common causes of swollen legs in the palliative care patient.

Unilateral:

- DVT
- Cellulitiis
- Nodal disease in groin
- Lymphoedema

Bilateral:

- DVT
- Hypoalbuminaemia
- Heart failure
- Medicines, for example, steroids, nifedipine
- Lymphoedema
- Pelvic disease causing reduced venous outflow

thromboprophylaxis based on recognized risk assessment models and would therefore require life-long prophylaxis.[55]

Revisiting the World Health Organization (WHO) definition of palliative care offers clarity to the way teams should manage the issue of thromboprophylaxis in the advanced cancer patient. A blanket thromboprophylaxis policy within the SPCU environment would be inappropriate, costly, and of no proven benefit. Palliative-care physicians, oncologists, intensive care physicians, and haematologists have differing views on which patients are appropriate for prophylaxis depending upon the clinical scenario but none would consider

Table 7.4 Common causes of dyspnoea in advanced cancer

- Pneumonia
- Pulmonary oedema
- Pleural effusion
- Anaemia
- Lung metastases
- Lymphangitis
- Muscle fatigue
- Concurrent pulmonary illness
  - COPD
  - Emphysema
  - Interstitial lung disease
  - Congestive cardiac failure

thromboprophylaxis appropriate in the last few days of life.[56] In considering thromboprophylaxis guidelines, one has a duty to protect the vulnerable whilst trying to help those who may benefit.

The WHO defines palliative care as aiming to 'neither to hasten or postpone death' but rather than taking it to be applied to the prolongation of the dying phase itself, some palliative physicians may feel uncomfortable with interventions perceived to be altering the natural history of the underlying disease. However, the definition also highlights the increasing emphasis to 'improve the quality of life of patients ... through the *prevention* and relief of suffering by means of early identification and *impeccable assessment* and treatment of pain and other problems'. There is an increasing understanding that palliative-care interventions such as good pain control, treatment of metabolic abnormalities, insertion of a ureteric stent, etc., can prolong survival and it may be increasingly challenging to judge whether an intervention is appropriate for an individual patient. Since prophylaxis protocols are generalized and do not focus specifically on palliative-care patients, there may be a temptation to ignore them as inappropriate for this patient group and hence also to ignore the VTE. Since the VTE risk is always present in advanced cancer patients, whether ambulant or hospitalized, one may be tempted to ignore the episodes when the thrombotic risk is temporarily increased further. A proportion of these patients may warrant consideration of prophylaxis. The WHO definition also highlights the need for a team approach to the management of patients and embraces the individualization of care. If one accepts that almost all SPCU inpatients will be at high risk of VTE and preventable VTE is likely to contribute to common and distressing symptoms, it would seem reasonable to consider the appropriateness of thromboprophylaxis on an individual patient basis. A team-based decision-making process, which considers the views of the patient lies at the heart of good palliative care and the prevention of VTE in a subgroup of palliative inpatients should be considered.

One suggested pathway, described below, has been developed specifically for the palliative-care setting and relies on a team decision following assessing the patient's general status, before considering the potential risks and possible benefits of thromboprophylaxis (Fig. 7.1). It also encourages these decisions to be reviewed on a regular basis.

Step 1: general assessment

The general assessment is to identify patients in whom thromboprophylaxis is clearly inappropriate, regardless of their risk of developing VTE. Thromboprophylaxis in a dying patient is universally considered to be inappropriate.[56] Dying patients are likely to develop VTE in the terminal stages as evidenced by postmortem studies, but these symptoms should be addressed with standard symptom control measures and end-of-life medicines.[57,58] Likewise, for patients admitted for anticipated terminal care and those considered unlikely to make any clinical improvement from their presentation could be managed symptomatically without thromboprophylaxis. There will be patients for whom thromboprophylaxis with LMWH is contraindicated such as those with a history of heparin-induced thrombocytopenia, active bleeding, or persistent thrombocytopenia, and those already anticoagulated who do not need another agent.

Step 2: risk assessment

As discussed previously, the presence of cancer is a recognized as an independent risk factor for VTE[5,6] and the NCCN guidelines,[7] Seventh ACCP guidelines,[8] and the latest IUA guidelines,[9] all categorize hospitalized cancer patients as a group at high or highest risk for VTE who should receive pharmacological thromboprophylaxis, unless contraindicated. Additional risk factors identified by the Thromboembolic Risk Factors (THRIFT) Consensus Group included immobility, age > 40, surgery, major medical illness including heart failure and infection, and recent trauma including acute SCI.[55] With respect to the palliative population, it is more important to identify whether there has been an acute event that has increased the thrombotic risk. Many patients may be immobile at home, yet do not receive thromboprophylaxis. It would seem counterintuitive to start such patients on LMWH when admitted to the SPCU unless there was a new additional risk factor. This is especially important in patients admitted for respite, where the clinical situation has not changed prior to admission.

Step 3: benefit assessment

Whilst the use of LMWH has not been formally assessed in the SPCU environment, there is a suggestion—from the evidence outlined in this chapter—that patients with reversible causes of acute deterioration may benefit from thromboprophylaxis. Since the evidence presented, albeit in a healthier population, shows a reduction in VTE, it may suggest that symptoms attributable to preventable VTE could be lessened. In addition, a proportion of patients, who until recently, enjoyed a good quality of life, may avoid a fatal PE at a time they are receiving treatment intended to return them to former well being.

Step 4: team decision

Palliative care teams frequently administer medicines off licence when the potential benefits outweigh the potential risks. Given the current evidence base, it is unlikely that many patients will be considered appropriate for thromboprophylaxis but in the small group that are appropriate, a team consensus is essential.

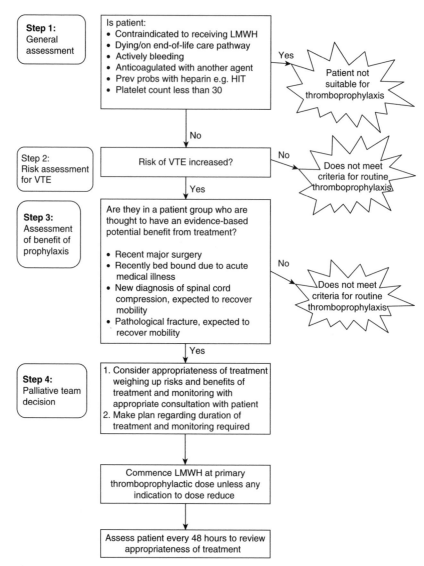

Fig. 7.1 Flow chart for consideration of primary prophylaxis for VTE in palliative patients.[(60)]

Conclusions

There is a strong theoretical argument for providing thromboprophylaxis to palliative-care inpatients, yet this is not supported by evidence in a representative population. However, absence of evidence should not be confused with absence of efficacy. A sufficiently powered RCT comparing thromboprophy-laxis with no thromboprophylaxis in palliative-care inpatients is warranted although careful identification of meaningful clinical endpoints is essential. A focus on quality of life and symptoms are of greater importance in these patients than survival and asymptomatic, radiologically proven VTE. In the meantime, an individualized approach to each patient would seem appropriate to identify those who may benefit from thromboprophylaxis as suggested by current evidence. Although this may be culturally challenging, it could be argued that a blanket policy to not give thromboprophylaxis is as ethically unacceptable as a policy that advocates thromboprophylaxis for all.

Case scenarios

Case 1: patient on the end-of-life care pathway

A 62-year-old lady with metastatic ovarian cancer and peritoneal involvement was admitted with abdominal pain, nausea, and vomiting. One week prior to admission, she had been self-caring but had taken to her bed because of her worsening symptoms. She was found to have multiple-level bowel obstruc-tion, which was not considered amenable for surgery. She was treated conservatively with a combination of steroids, parenteral antiemetics, and analgesics given via a syringe driver. Her symptoms improved on a combina-tion of octreotide and levomepromazine but her overall condition deteriorated and she was commenced on the local hospital end-of-life care pathway. On admission, she had been started on prophylactic LMWH, which has continued to this point.

The initial decision to commence thromboprophylaxis would have been appropriate since the patient on admission has potentially reversible cause for her deterioration and had been well prior to the acute events leading to her admission. She had multiple risk factors for VTE, including recent immobility and advanced malignancy. This case illustrates the importance of regular assessment and review of the need to consider thromboprophylaxis. Her changing condition and imminent death quite rightly call into question the indication of LMWH at this stage. It is normal practice to rationalize the medicines as someone enters the terminal phase to essential drugs only. LMWH is unlikely to offer any benefit to the patient's terminal care, and symptoms attributable to VTE can be adequately managed with appropriate end-of-life drugs.

Case 2: patient with chronic lung disease, acute pneumonia, and hypercalcaemia

A 70-year-old man has recently been diagnosed with stage IIIb non-small-cell lung cancer (T4 N2 M0). He has advanced chronic obstructive pulmonary disease (COPD) and was considered unfit for palliative chemotherapy. The cancer was picked up on an X-ray following a recent admission for pneumonia. He lives alone but remains self-caring with no additional support. His daughter lived nearby and visits daily. He has no specific symptoms from his lung cancer.

He is admitted with a further infective exacerbation of his COPD and commenced on intravenous antibiotics. He is found to be hypercalcaemic and receives fluids and bisphosphonates.

> This man has been self-caring and is now admitted with an acute deterioration. Additional to his malignancy, he has new risk factors for VTE namely pneumonia, immobility, and dehydration. All these are potentially reversible and the team has made a decision to treat these. It would be appropriate to commence LMWH prophylaxis until he is discharged home.

Case 3: acute SCC

A 56-year-old lady with metastatic breast cancer is admitted from clinic with back pain and right leg weakness. Clinical suspicion of acute SCC is confirmed by magnetic resonance imaging (MRI), which shows multiple levels of compression from metastatic deposits in the thoracic vertebrae. There is evidence of vertebral collapse, consistent with her back pain and neurology. She is admitted and given high-dose dexamethasone and a 5-day course of radiotherapy. She is initially nursed flat, then subsequently sat up, and rehabilitated according to local guidelines.

> Acute SCC is one of the most thrombogenic clinical scenarios faced by patients with advanced cancer. This patient has an ongoing VTE risk due to metastatic malignancy, which has been acutely raised by vertebral collapse from bone metastases and subsequent immobilization for radiotherapy and rehabilitation. Without thromboprophylaxis she is at high risk of VTE. This lady was mobile at the time of admission and is likely to be discharged home with minimal neurological deficit. LMWH prophylaxis would be indicated until discharge.

Case 4: respite admission

A 63-year-old man with advanced motor neuron disease is admitted to the hospice for 2 weeks respite for his wife, the main carer. His condition has deteriorated over the past 3 months and he is now bedbound and dependant on full nursing care. Despite his deterioration, he is able to communicate effectively and enjoys what he describes as 'an acceptable quality of life'.

This man has been immobile for some time without prophylaxis and the prothrombotic risk had not altered from his planned admission. He has no acute episodes that may alter his thrombotic risk and he has been clinically symptom free of VTE in his usual place of care. Little would be gained from giving LMWH in this situation. If he were to develop pneumonia whilst in hospital and the team decision to treat this acute infection was made, thromboprophylaxis should then be considered and discussed with the patient.

Key points

- The majority of evidence supporting thromboprophylaxis in the palliative setting is extrapolated from general medical and surgical populations.
- The heterogeneity of the palliative-care population makes it difficult to produce 'one size fits all' guidelines.
- Thromboprophylaxis is inappropriate in the terminal phases since symptoms attributable to VTE can be managed with end-of-life drugs.
- Cancer patients admitted with reversible causes for acute deterioration should be considered for thromboprophylaxis until the acute event has resolved.
- Decisions should be made by the team on an individual patient basis, taking account of a patient's wishes.
- Thromboprophylaxis decisions should be reviewed regularly.

References

1. Noble SIR, Hood K, Finlay IG. Have palliative care teams' attitudes toward venous thromboembolism changed? A survey of thromboprophylaxis practice across British specialist palliative care units in the years 2000 and 2005. *Journal of Pain and Symptom Management* 2006;32(1):38–43.

2. Geerts WH, Pineo GF, Heit JA *et al.* Prevention of venous thromboembolism: the Seventh ACCP Conference on Antithrombotic and Thrombolytic Therapy. *Chest* 2004 Sep;126(3 Suppl):338S–400S

3. Cohen AT, Tapson VF, Bergmann JF *et al.* Venous thromboembolism risk and prophylaxis in the acute hospital care setting (ENDORSE study): a multinational cross-sectional study. *Lancet* 2008;2;371(9610):387–94.

4. Tapson VF, Decousus H, Pini M *et al.* Venous thromboembolism prophylaxis in acutely ill hospitalized medical patients: findings from the International Medical Prevention Registry on Venous Thromboembolism. *Chest* 2007 Sep;132(3):936–45.

5. Heit JA, Silverstein MD, Mohr DN *et al.* Risk factors for deep vein thrombosis and pulmonary embolism: a population-based case-control study. *Archives of Internal Medicine* 2000;160:809–15.

6. Alikhan R, Cohen AT, Combe S *et al.* MEDENOX Study. Risk factors for venous thromboembolism in hospitalized patients with acute medical illness: analysis of the MEDENOX Study. *Archives of Internal Medicine* 2004;164:963–8.

7. Khorana AA. The NCCN clinical practice guidelines on venous thromboembolic disease: strategies for improving VTE prophylaxis in hospitalized cancer patients. *The Oncologist* 2007 Nov;12(11):1361–70.

8. Snow V, Qaseem A, Barry P *et al.* American College of Physicians; American Academy of Family Physicians Panel on Deep Venous Thrombosis/Pulmonary Embolism. Management of venous thromboembolism: a clinical practice guideline from the American College of Physicians and the American Academy of Family Physicians. *Annals of Internal Medicine* 2007;146:204–10.

9. Cardiovascular Disease Educational and Research Trust; Cyprus Cardiovascular Disease Educational and Research Trust; European Venous Forum; International Surgical Thrombosis Forum; International Union of Angiology; Union Internationale de Phlebologie. Prevention and treatment of venous thromboembolism. International Consensus Statement (guidelines according to scientific evidence). *International Angiology* 2006;25:101–61.

10. Kirwan CC, Nath E, Byrne GJ *et al.* Prophylaxis for venous thromboembolism during treatment for cancer: questionnaire survey. *British Medical Journal* 2003;13;327(7415):597–8.

11. Burleigh E, Wang C, Foster D *et al.* Thromboprophylaxis in medically ill patients at risk for venous thromboembolism. *American Journal of Health-System Pharmacy* 2006;63(suppl 6):S23–9

12. Kakkar AK, Levine M, Pinedo HM *et al.* Venous thrombosis in cancer patients: insights from the FRONTLINE survey. *The Oncologist* 2003;8(4):381–8.

13. Kahn SR, Panju A, Geerts W *et al.* CURVE study investigators. Multicenter evaluation of the use of venous thromboembolism prophylaxis in acutely ill medical patients in Canada. *Thrombosis Research* 2007;119:145–55.

14. Geerts WH, Heit JA, Clagett GP *et al.* Prevention of venous thromboembolism. *Chest* 2001;119:132S–75S.

15. Wells PS, Lensing AW, Hirsh J. Graduated compression stockings in the prevention of postoperative venous thromboembolism: a meta-analysis. *Archives of Internal Medicine* 1994;154:67–72.

16. Mismetti P, Laporte S, Darmon JY *et al*. Meta-analysis of low molecular weight heparin in the prevention of venous thromboembolism in general surgery. *British Journal of Surgery* 2001;88:913–30.

17. ENOXACAN Study Group. Efficacy and safety of enoxaparin versus unfractionated heparin for prevention of deep vein thrombosis in elective cancer surgery: a double-blind randomized multicentre trial with venographic assessment. ENOXACAN Study Group. *British Journal of Surgery* 1997;84:1099–103.

18. Bergqvist D, Agnelli G, Cohen AT *et al*. Duration of prophylaxis against venous thromboembolism with enoxaparin after surgery for cancer. *The New England Journal of Medicine* 2002;346(13):975–80.

19. Agnelli G, Bergqvist D, Cohen AT *et al*. Randomized clinical trial of postoperative fondaparinux versus perioperative dalteparin for prevention of venous thromboembolism in high-risk abdominal surgery. *British Journal of Surgery* 2005;92(10):1212–20.

20. Clarke-Pearson DL, Coleman RE, Synan IS *et al*. Venous thromboembolism prophylaxis in gynecologic oncology: a prospective, controlled trial of low-dose heparin. *American Journal of Obstetrics and Gynecology* 1983;145:606–13.

21. Clarke-Pearson DL, Creasman WT, Coleman RE *et al*. Perioperative external pneumatic calf compression as thromboembolism prophylaxis in gynecologic oncology: report of a randomized controlled trial. *Gynecologic Oncology* 1984;18:226–32.

22. Fricker JP, Vergnes Y, Schach R *et al*. Low dose heparin versus low molecular weight heparin (Kabi 2165, Fragmin) in the prophylaxis of thromboembolic complications of abdominal oncological surgery. *European Journal of Clinical Investigation* 1988;18:561–7.

23. von Tempelhoff GF, Dietrich M, Niemann F *et al*. Blood coagulation and thrombosis in patients with ovarian malignancy. *Thrombosis and Haemostasis* 1997;77:456–61.

24. Clarke-Pearson DL, DeLong E, Synan IS *et al*. A controlled trial of two low-dose heparin regimens for the prevention of postoperative deep vein thrombosis. *Obstetrics and Gynecology* 1990;75:684–9.

25. Heilmann L, von Tempelhoff GF, Kirkpatrick C *et al*. Comparison of unfractionated versus low molecular weight heparin for deep vein thrombosis prophylaxis during breast and pelvic cancer surgery: efficacy, safety, and follow-up. *Clinical and Applied Thrombosis/Hemostasis* 1998;4:268–73.

26. Baykal C, Al A, Demirtas E *et al*. Comparison of enoxaparin and standard heparin in gynaecologic oncologic surgery: a randomised prospective double-blind clinical study. *European Journal of Gynaecological Oncology* 2001;22:127–30.

27. Oates-Whitehead RM, D'Angelo A, Mol B. Anticoagulant and aspirin prophylaxis for preventing thromboembolism after major gynaecological surgery. *Cochrane Database of Systematic Reviews* 2003;4:CD003679.

28. Semrad TJ, O'Donnell R, Wun T *et al*. Epidemiology of venous thromboembolism in 9489 patients with malignant glioma. *Journal of Neurosurgery* 2007;106(4):601–8.

29. Marras LC, Geerts WH, Perry JR. The risk of venous thromboembolism is increased throughout the course of malignant glioma: an evidence-based review. *Cancer* 2000;89:640–6.

30. Nurmohamed MT, van Riel AM, Henkens CM *et al.* Low molecular weight heparin and compression stockings in the prevention of venous thromboembolism in neurosurgery. *Thrombosis and Haemostasis* 1996;75:233–8.

31. Agnelli G, Piovella F, Buoncristiani P *et al.* Enoxaparin plus compression stockings compared with compression stockings alone in the prevention of venous thromboembolism after elective neurosurgery. *The New England Journal of Medicine* 1998;339:80–5.

32. Iorio A, Agnelli G. Low-molecular-weight and unfractionated heparin for prevention of venous thromboembolism in neurosurgery: a meta-analysis. *Archives of Internal Medicine* 2000;160:2327–32.

33. Kramer J. Spinal cord compression in malignancy. *Palliative Medicine* 1992;6:202–11.

34. Cowap J, Hardy JR. A'Hern ROutcome of malignant spinal cord compression at a cancer center: implications for palliative care services. *Journal of Pain and Symptom Management* Apr 2000;19(4):257–64.

35. Waring WP, Karunas RS. Acute spinal cord injuries and the incidence of clinically occuring thromboembolic disease. *Paraplegia* 1991;29:8–16.

36. Kim SW, Charallel JT, Park KW *et al.* Prevalence of deep venous thrombosis in patients with chronic spinal cord injury. *Archives of Physical Medicine and Rehabilitation* 1994;75:965–8.

37. DeVivo MJ, Krause JS, Lammertse DP. Recent trends in mortality and causes of death among persons with spinal cord injury. *Archives of Physical Medicine and Rehabilitation* 1999;80:1411–9.

38. Spinal Cord Injury Thromboprophylaxis Investigators. Prevention of venous thromboembolism in the acute treatment phase after spinal cord injury: a randomized, multicenter trial comparing low-dose heparin plus intermittent pneumatic compression with enoxaparin. *The Journal of Trauma* 2003;54:1116–26.

39. Heit JA, Silverstein MD, Mohr DN *et al.* Risk factors for deep vein thrombosis and pulmonary embolism: a population-based case-control study. *Archives of Internal Medicine* 2000;160:809–15.

40. Samama MM, Cohen AT, Darmon JY *et al.* A comparison of enoxaparin with placebo for the prevention of venous thromboembolism in acutely ill medical patients. Prophylaxis in Medical Patients with Enoxaparin Study Group. *The New England Journal of Medicine* 1999;341:793–800.

41. Leizorovicz A, Cohen AT, Turpie AG *et al.* PREVENT Medical Thromboprophylaxis Study Group. Randomized, placebo-controlled trial of dalteparin for the prevention of venous thromboembolism in acutely ill medical patients. *Circulation* 2004;110:874–9.

42. Mismetti P, Laporte-Simitsidis S, Tardy B *et al.* Prevention of venous thromboembolism in internal medicine with unfractionated or low-molecular-weight heparins: a meta-analysis of randomised clinical trials. *Thrombosis and Haemostasis* 2000;83:14–9.

43. Cohen AT, Davidson BL, Gallus AS *et al.* Efficacy and safety of fondaparinux for the prevention of venous thromboembolism in older acute medical patients: randomised placebo controlled trial. *British Medical Journal* 2006; 332:325–9.

44. Levine M, Hirsh J, Gent M *et al.* Double-blind randomised trial of a very-low-dose warfarin for prevention of thromboembolism in stage IV breast cancer. *Lancet* 1994;343(8902):886–9.

45. Zonder JA. Thrombotic complications of myeloma therapy. *Hematology American Society of Hematology Education Book.* 2006;348–55.

46. Palumbo A, Rajkumar SV, Dimopoulos MA *et al.* Prevention of thalidomide- and lenalidomide-associated thrombosis in myeloma. *Leukemia* 2008;22(2):414–23.

47. Noble SI, Nelson A, Turner C *et al.* Acceptability of low molecular weight heparin thromboprophylaxis for inpatients receiving palliative care: qualitative study. *British Medical Journal* 2006;332(7541):577–80.

48. Chambers JC. Prophylactic heparin in palliative care: … to a challenging idea. *British Medical Journal* 2006;332(7543):729.

49. World Health Organization. *Definition of palliative care.* www.who.int/cancer/palliative/definition/en/ (accessed 12th Feb 2008).

50. Prandoni P, Lensing AW, Piccioli A *et al.* Recurrent venous thromboembolism and bleeding complications during anticoagulant treatment in patients with cancer and venous thrombosis. *Blood* 2002;100(10):3484–8.

51. Noble S. The challenges of managing cancer related venous thromboembolism in the palliative care setting. *Postgraduate Medical Journal* 2007 Nov;83(985):671–4.

52. Johnson MJ, Sherry K. How do palliative physicians manage venous thromboembolism? *Palliative Medicine* 1997 Nov;11(6):462–8.

53. Johnson MJ, Sproule MW, Paul J. The prevalence and associated variables of deep venous thrombosis in patients with advanced cancer. *Clinical oncology* (Royal College of Radiologists (Great Britain)) 1999;11(2):105–10.

54. Johnson MJ, Chapter 5. Management of VTE in a palliative care setting. In MD thesis: *Venous thromboembolism in advanced cancer.* University of Manchester 1999 pp.134–7.

55. Thromboembolic Risk Factors (THRIFT) Consensus Group. Risk of and prophylaxis for venous thromboembolism in hospital patients. *British Medical Journal* 1992;305:567–74.

56. Kierner KA, Gartner V, Schwarz M *et al.* Use of thromboprophylaxis in palliative care patients: a survey among experts in palliative care, oncology, intensive care, and anticoagulation. *The American Journal of Hospice and Palliative Care* 2008;25(2):127–31.

57. Sproul EE. Carcinoma and venous thrombosis: the frequency of association of carcinoma in the body or tail of the pancreas with multiple venous thrombosis. *The American Journal of Cancer* 1938;34:566–85.

58. Ambrus JL, Ambrus CM, Pickren JW. Causes of death in cancer patients. *Journal of Medicine* 1975;6:61–4.

59. O'Doherty CA, Hall EJ, Schofield L *et al.* Drugs and syringe drivers: a survey of adult specialist palliative care practice in the United Kingdom and Eire. *Palliative Medicine* 2001 Mar;15(2):149–54.

60. Aslett M, Lock A. Guidelines and evidence: primary prophylaxis for venous thromboembolism (VTE) in palliative patients with malignancy. 2008. *Pan Birmingham End of Life Network.*

Chapter 8

Clinical decision-making: treatment of venous thromboembolism in patients with advanced cancer

Dawn Dowding and Miriam J. Johnson

Introduction

The decision to treat a patient having venous thromboembolism (VTE) with anticoagulation is one based on a large body of evidence. Anticoagulation first with low molecular weight heparin (LMWH) and then an oral coumarin therapy is an established medical practice. Likewise, the length of time required for anticoagulation for a deep vein thrombosis (DVT) or pulmonary embolism (PE) is set into clinical guidelines. However, when the clinician is faced with a patient with advanced cancer—who has developed a VTE—the decision-making is not as straightforward because of the challenges outlined in Chapter 1. In this chapter, we consider specific issues connected with deciding on whether or not to treat a patient with VTE in the palliative-care setting. We then consider how strategies from the broader literature on decision-making in healthcare could be applied to the palliative-care setting, in order to assist clinicians with this difficult area of practice.

Issues in the palliative-care setting

Despite the long recognized association between cancer and VTE and increasing understanding of the underlying pathophysiology, it can still be difficult to know how best to manage the patient in the palliative setting, particularly where the patient is not imminently dying of their disease (Fig. 8.1). Specific problems are outlined in Box 8.1 and discussed more fully in Chapter 1. Factors that may influence treatment decision-making include the inherent risks associated with treating VTE, costs of therapy, and clinicians' own knowledge and attitudes towards decision-making (Table 8.1).

Box 8.1 Specific problems in the palliative-care setting

- Increased risk of bleeding—both due to tumour and due to anticoagulation—and an increased risk of recurrence despite adequate anticoagulation.
- Difficulties in weighing up the relative burdens and benefits of anticoagulation in a patient of reduced performance status, quality of life, and prognosis.
- Practical issues around administering and monitoring anticoagulation, venous access problems, and issues around long-term parenteral administration of LMWH.
- Difficulties in estimating prognosis.
- Complications related to the tumour or its treatment, which impact on the risk of anticoagulation such as thrombocytopenia or brain metastases.
- Little directly applicable evidence to inform the clinician. Much of the research has been done on patients who are less unwell than our patient group, and is therefore not straightforward to apply and much is still unknown.
- Clinicians not all aware of specific issues in cancer patients, particularly in generalist fields.

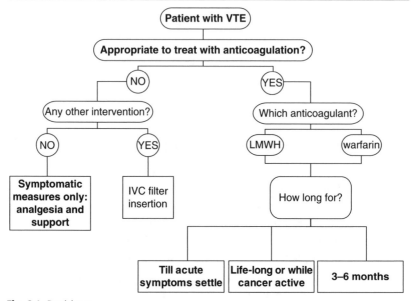

Fig. 8.1 Decisions.

Table 8.1 Factors that influence decision steps.

Decision	Factors influencing
To be anticoagulated or not	Disease factors; mild, moderate, extensive; thrombocytopenia, brain metastases; genito-urinary, gastro-intestinal primary site
	Patient factors; choice influenced by previous experience, goals (e.g., forthcoming family wedding), fear of bleeding/needles
	Treatment factors; availability of IVC filter service; local drug and therapeutic policies re LMWH
	Clinician factors; previous experience, knowledge, paternalism
If not for anticoagulation, IVC filter or not	Disease factors; high risk of bleeding or current bleeding; tumour masses causing technical difficulty in insertion
	Patient factors; willingness to undergo a procedure; fitness to tolerate procedure
	Treatment factors; availability and access to service
	Clinician factors; conflicting evidence as to benefit/risks
Which anticoagulant?	Similar to above
How long to anticoagulate?	Benefit/burden balance of treatment taking into account patient wishes. This balance will alter as the disease progresses and will be influenced by many of the issues tabled above

Risks and benefits of management

This is considered more fully in Chapter 6. However, we have summarized the key issues here to illustrate the complexity of decision-making surrounding this area. It has been identified that the disseminated intravascular coagulation caused by factors secreted by the tumour cells worsens with increasing tumour activity (see Chapter 3). Therefore, it is not surprising that in Prandoni's prospective observational cohort, patients with more extensive disease had a higher hazard ratio for both recurrent clotting and bleeding risk than for those with less-extensive disease.[1]

There are also many features that make treatment with anticoagulants hazardous, with patients at increased risk both of clotting and bleeding compared with patients with nonmalignant disease and VTE. Thus, it can be difficult to know how best to treat patients in practice, particularly those with moderate or extensive disease. There is some evidence that standard anticoagulant regimens with oral warfarin in cancer patients with VTE is less effective and higher risk than long-term LMWH, and some evidence that inferior vena caval filters may be of benefit to some patients although other authors suggest filters are not appropriate in patients with advanced cancer (see Chapter 6). There is little to guide the clinician in the patient with advanced disease or where particular situations give a cause for concern such as the presence of intracranial tumour, or an already bleeding lesion. Monreal's prospective study in patients with advanced disease indicates that a reduced dose regimen of LMWH may be as effective.[2]

Costs of therapy

Cost of drug does have an influence, and warfarin is very cheap compared with LMWH. Although it could be argued that prevention of even one anticoagulant-related complication or recurrent thrombosis resulting in hospital admission renders LMWH more cost-effective, the clinicians and managers have pressures to keep drug costs down, which may influence some.

Currently, LMWH is not licensed in the UK for long-term administration although it is in the US for cancer patients with VTE. Despite this, their use in this manner is becoming a standard practice in obstetrics and now incorporated into cancer-related VTE treatment guidelines. Clinicians who are unfamiliar with LMWH, or who do not understand the issues relating to licensing, misinterpreting 'unlicensed indication' as 'not permitted' may be reluctant to prescribe in this way.

Clinicians' knowledge

Decisions may be influenced more by 'last bad experience' or lack of, than evidence-based thought. Existing literature has highlighted that even when clinicians have knowledge of research evidence, this is rarely enough by itself to change practice.[3] There is a further risk that clinicians may use what may be conflicting evidence to suit their own management preferences, even if they are skilled at critical appraisal of literature.

Decision-making and treatment of VTE in patients with cancer

There has been limited research into how clinicians make decisions regarding whether or not to use anticoagulation therapy in patients with cancer and VTE. Studies exist that have focused on ways of identifying individuals who are *at risk* of developing a VTE, in order to provide preventative anticoagulation therapy.[4,5] In these studies, the presence of malignancy has been identified as a high risk factor, thereby indicating that anticoagulation therapy should be considered.[4,5] A study comparing competing guidelines for the administration of prophylactic heparin treatment found that there was moderate agreement within the four guidelines assessed to recommend prophylactic treatment in patients who had malignancy and one or more additional risk factors (e.g., bedridden).[6] There is evidence that palliative physicians find treatment of VTE in patients with advanced cancer difficult and may be reluctant to investigate or treat.[7] If treatment is instigated, then sub-therapeutic regimens may be used, thus leaving the patient in double jeopardy of increased risk of bleeding and a less-effective secondary prevention.

Although difficult to find other than anecdotally, there is a perception that patients in the palliative setting should not be treated for VTE because 'a nice big PE is a good way to go'. However, postmortem evidence suggests that a PE is not necessarily 'a nice way to go'; 25 per cent of patients taking over an hour to die rather than immediately, with two-thirds of the abruptly dead having symptoms of 'advertising emboli'. Thus, even fatal PE may be the cause of considerable morbidity, that is, potentially preventable or treatable.[8] Also, even in the event of a 'nice big PE', it may not have been the patient's choice to die suddenly, often in an undignified manner, for example, on the toilet, and this may also have implications for the bereaved. In a recent study, Noble *et al.* have demonstrated that patients wish to be included in treatment decisions and not treated with clinical paternalism with this regard, at least with VTE prophylaxis.[9]

Summary

It is not known how UK oncologists, palliative physicians, or general practitioners (all of whom may be involved in the care of patients with advanced cancer) come to clinical decisions regarding the management of VTE in patients with advanced noncurative cancer, and it is likely that there is little consistency between or within the different groups. Clinicians appear to find decision-making surrounding the management of patients with cancer and VTE difficult. This is unsurprising given the complexity of the treatment management decisions that they face. Recent research has suggested that patients would welcome being involved in such treatment decision-making. The rest of this chapter explores approaches to clinical decision-making from the broader medical literature, which may assist clinicians when faced with such complex clinical situations.

Decision-making in healthcare

Decision-making in healthcare often operates under conditions of uncertainty, where it is unclear what is actually wrong with the patient, or which treatment may be appropriate for that patient. This can lead to variations in how clinicians make decisions, and subsequently variations in the care that patients receive.[10] While making treatment decisions, clinicians often use a process of '*ad hoc*' decision-making, where they use some form of global judgement about what might be the best course of action for that patient.[11] These *ad hoc* decisions may be based on a number of factors, such as what a clinician has been taught, their clinical experience of other patients with that particular disease/condition, or what is common practice within their particular institution.[11] This may lead to patients being treated inappropriately, as a number of studies have highlighted clinicians' judgements and decisions may be governed by heuristics or bias, which may lead to errors in their decision-making. Heuristics are cognitive processes or 'rules of thumb' commonly used by humans when making decisions, which are used unconsciously, but may lead to mistakes.[12]

Examples of such heuristics (see Table 8.2) include *representativeness*, where judgements of the likelihood of an event occurring are based on how closely it

Table 8.2 Common heuristics.

Availability	The probability of an event is estimated based on how easily an individual can recall a similar event from their memory. For instance, a doctor judges the patient has a particular disease because their case reminds them of a similar vivid case they have recently seen. This can lead to errors, as individuals often recall recent or vivid events more easily, rather than considering the actual likelihood of an event in the wider population.
Representativeness	The probability of an event is estimated based on how similar (or representative) it is of a wider category of events. For instance, a doctor judges a patient has a particular disease because the patient's signs and symptoms are 'representative' of that disease. It can lead to errors such as the neglect of the base rate of the disease in a specific patient population.
Anchoring and adjustment	The probability of an event is estimated by taking an initial reference point (anchor) and then adjusting this to reach a final judgement about the likelihood. For instance, a doctor judges the likelihood of the patient having a particular disease is 60 per cent. They collect information (perhaps from diagnostic tests) and reassess their estimation on the basis of these results to come to a final diagnosis. It can lead to errors, as final estimations of likelihood are linked to the original anchor—so if this is highly inaccurate, the final judgement is also likely to be inaccurate.

resembles other similar events; *availability*, where judgements of the likelihood of an event are based on how easily similar events are remembered; and *anchoring and adjustment*, where assessments of the likelihood of an event are anchored on an initial estimate and then adjusted to take into account the individual features of the patient.[12–14] Other factors that may also influence clinicians' decisions include *framing effects*, where how different treatment options are presented to a decision maker (for instance, in terms of the likely amount of lives gained or the number of lives lost) affects the decision an individual makes.[15–17]

There are ways in which clinicians can avoid the pitfalls of using *ad hoc*, unconscious decision processes to make decisions about patient care. Evidence-based medicine (EBM) suggests that decisions about patient treatment should be made based on 'the integration of best research evidence with clinical expertise and patient values'[18] (p.1). By ensuring that treatment decisions are based on research evidence, it is assumed that the decisions taken will be more informed and therefore better for patients. However, one key issue in the practice of EBM is *how* to integrate research evidence about both the benefits and risks of different treatment options, with patient preferences for those options, in a way that helps to inform decision-making.

One approach that has been suggested as a way of tackling this issue is through the use of decision analysis.[19–22] Decision analysis is a quantitative approach to structuring decisions, which models the decision problem in the form of decision trees. The likelihood or probability of uncertain events occurring is then added to the tree, where the probabilities are identified from high-quality research studies (where available). The value or preference patients attach to different treatment options/outcomes is also assessed numerically (known as patient utility). Both probabilities and utilities are then used to calculate the optimum option for the decision being modelled (known as maximizing expected utility), with the preferred option being the one that has the highest value.[20,23]

Clinical decision analysis has previously been used to determine the optimal strategy for managing and preventing VTE in cancer-related hypercoagulable states.[24] The model considered the consequences of bleeding and thromboembolic events, filter complications, and cancer-excess mortality on quality-adjusted life expectancy and average costs. Data was drawn from the current literature at that time. They concluded that filter placement and long-term oral anticoagulant therapy resulted in similar outcomes, but that filter insertion was cheaper. Since then, however, we now have randomized controlled trial data in support of long-term LMWH, and still have little understanding of the role of filter placement in advanced cancer patients. The conclusions are therefore likely to be different if repeated.

Clinical decision analysis has also been used to assist clinicians make decisions about anticoagulation for patients with atrial fibrillation (AF), where the issues of competing risks and benefits of treatment, and the importance of patient preferences/values are similar to the treatment decision issues highlighted in this chapter.[25,26] Evaluating patients' preferences for different treatment options is important in such complex decisions, as patients' preferences often differ to the recommendations from clinical guidelines.[27,28] The models from clinical decision analysis have also been used to inform decision aids, which can be used by clinicians and patients to assist with the decision-making process, regarding whether or not to recommend anticoagulation therapy for AF.[29] Clinical decision analysis may therefore have the potential to help clinicians and patients with cancer make a decision about whether or not anticoagulation therapy is appropriate for their individual case. Examples of how this approach may be used for patients with advanced cancer and VTE can be seen in Case Scenario 1.

Case scenarios

Case 1

A 68-year-old single lady with endometrial carcinoma; mild but continuous bleeding PV, coping but feels she wouldn't cope if it got any worse. She presents with a 3-month history of progressive breathlessness such that she now cannot walk across her small lounge to the bathroom without severe breathlessness. A ventilation-perfusion scan shows multiple PE. In this instance, the decision-making problem is whether or not to use LMWH or warfarin for anticoagulation, insert a filter, or do nothing.

As an exercise to show the process of decision analysis, Table 8.3 uses an approximation of likelihood of outcomes from relevant literature and potential utility values (patient preferences) for each of the options, based on the assumptions of the clinician involved. This is not intended to be exhaustive, indeed it is difficult to extrapolate relevant occurrence probabilities and it is acknowledged that bleeding and recurrent clotting are not mutually exclusive. However, it is included in Table 8.3 to illustrate the process that might be used.

What are patient utilities?

Utility values are a measure of the value that an individual (or group of individuals) places on the different outcomes of a decision.[30] It may also be known as a 'health state preference' and is not the same as quality of life measures, which focus on the *characteristics* of a health state, rather than the

Table 8.3 Outcomes and utilities of different treatment options.

Intervention	Potential outcomes	Probability of occurrence	Utility of outcome
Anticoagulation with warfarin	Bleeding gets worse (any bleeding–major bleeding)	16.5 per cent (average of [32,33] – average major bleed)	0
	Major bleed	5.5 per cent over 3 months[1] (genito-urinary tumour = 4.5 hazard ratio of non cancer)	0
	Recurrent thrombosis	16 per cent[33,34]	20
	Symptoms resolve	62 per cent[33,34] – assuming bleeding and thrombosis are mutually exclusive	100
Anticoagulation with fixed reduced-dose LMWH	Bleeding gets worse (any bleeding)	7.9–5.4 = 2.5 per cent over 3 months[2] (fixed-dose LMWH)	0
	Major bleed	5.4 per cent over 3 months[2] (fixed-dose LMWH)	0
	Recurrent thrombosis	8.9 per cent[2] (fixed-dose LMWH)	20
	Symptoms resolve	83.2 per cent (assuming bleed and clot are mutually exclusive)	100
Filter insertion	Death from procedure	0.5 per cent[24]	0
	PE	1 – 2.5; median 1.5 per cent	0
	Symptomatic recurrent/extending DVT	15 per cent[35]	20
	Symptoms resolve	83 per cent	100
No anticoagulation or filter	Symptoms worse with continuous VTE	40 per cent[32]	20
	Fatal PE	Sarasin[24] uses 50–60 per cent in his model but this is based on post mortem findings and it is therefore difficult to extrapolate that the PEs found were the cause of death, but use with reservations	0
	Symptoms resolve	10 per cent	100

value or preference attached to it.[31] Utility measures can be obtained in a number of ways and are commonly measured on a scale from 0 to 100, with 0 representing the worst possible outcome for an individual and 100 representing the best.

Carrying out a decision analysis

These values can be placed into a decision analysis model (shown in Fig. 8.2). The decision problem is represented as a decision tree, with the different options available as branches in the tree. Off each of the branches are the possible outcomes that could occur if you choose the option, with the probability or likelihood of that occurring. The utility values for each outcome are given at the end of the branch.

The decision analysis is calculated by 'folding back' the tree; the probability for each outcome is multiplied with its utility value, then the value for each outcome is added together to give a value for each decision option.

For example, for the 'anticoagulate with warfarin' branch:

$$(0.165 \times 0) + (0.055 \times 0) + (0.160 \times 20) + (0.620 \times 100) = 0 + 0 + 3.2 + 62 = 65.2$$

Decision analysis works on the assumption that a decision maker is logical and rational. Therefore, the branch with the highest overall value once each branch has been calculated (the option with the highest *expected utility*) is the

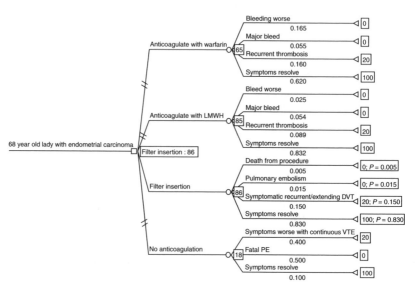

Fig. 8.2 Decision analysis for Case 1.

option that the decision maker should use. A summary of the overall values for each option in this model is as follows:

Anticoagulate with warfarin = 65

Anticoagulate with LMWH = 85

Filter insertion = 86

No anticoagulation = 18

In this example, using the values given in Table 8.3, the best option for this patient would be to do a filter insertion, as this is the option with the highest value (and therefore the highest expected utility). However, the value for anticoagulation with LMWH is close to that of filter insertion (85 opposed to 86) indicating that the decision is very close and is likely to be dependent upon the values that the patient associates with the different outcomes; in this case, the patient's preference not to allow any increased risk of bleeding. If the utility values in the analysis are altered, this may change the optimum treatment option. Decision analysis therefore reflects both the research evidence available for the decision and the variation in preferences that may occur between patients.

Case 2

A 35-year-old man with primary brain tumour with still good performance status develops a big left femoral DVT, which means he can no longer walk due to pain, heaviness, and swelling of his leg. He has two children at home aged six and eight and he wishes to stay at home if possible.

Decisions to make and issues to take into account:

- ◆ Which treatment option is most appropriate to someone who does not want hospital admission: filter, anticoagulation with warfarin or anticoagulation with LMWH, or general symptomatic measures only?

- ◆ Should he be investigated or his likely DVT treated empirically, bearing in mind that he lives in a rural area, now cannot drive and is worried about who would look after his children?

- ◆ His previous good performance status and child care role are important features that make the risk of a PE more clinically significant—his wish is to stay home to care for his children for as long as possible.

- ◆ The site of his tumour makes the risk of an anticoagulant-related bleed more clinically significant.

Case 3

A 52-year-old lady with sigmoid cancer has had her third-line chemotherapy stopped midcourse because of disease progression and persistent poor marrow reserve. (Platelet count $<20 \times 10^{-9}$/L) She developed bowel obstruction and undergoes a defunctioning colostomy with platelet infusion cover. Postoperatively, she develops large right femoral DVT. Three days later, she had an episode of breathlessness, which she found frightening, but which settled after about 2 hours leaving her with some residual breathless on effort. Her daughter is getting married in 4 weeks time.

> Decisions to make and issues to take into account:
>
> - Anticoagulate or not?
> - She has a likely short prognosis; therefore a filter is not an option.
> - Both the symptoms and her short-term goal (daughter's wedding) gives weight to call for at least short-term anticoagulation.
> - Low platelet count increases risk of bleeding with anticoagulation.
> - Monreal's study[2] suggests his fixed low-dose regimen may be appropriate.
> - What is the risk/benefit balance of anticoagulation in her opinion?

Conclusion

In this chapter, we have outlined the complexities of decision-making for clinicians when faced with a patient with cancer and VTE. Despite evidence of the benefits of LMWH for such patients, clinicians need to also consider the patient's wishes, which may include being involved in the decision-making process. Clinical decision analysis is a tool available to clinicians, which can integrate both research evidence and measures of patient preferences (in the form of utility measurements) in order to suggest what the optimum option may be for that patient. It is a useful tool for complex and uncertain decisions. However, its utility for this specific type of decision problem needs to be investigated further.

References

1. Prandoni P, Lensing A, Piccioli A *et al.* Recurrent venous thromboembolism and bleeding complications during anticoagulant treatment in patients with cancer and venous thrombosis. *Blood* 2002;100(10):3484–8.
2. Monreal M, Zacharski L, Jimenez J *et al.* Fixed-dose low-molecular-weight heparin for secondary prevention of venous thromboembolism in patients with disseminated cancer: a prospective cohort study. *Journal of Thrombosis and Haemostasis* 2004;2:1311–5.

3. Centre for Reviews and Dissemination. Getting Evidence into Practice. Effective *HealthCare* 1999;5(1):1–16.

4. Samama M, Dahl O, Mismetti P *et al.* An electronic tool for venous thromboembolism prevention in medical and surgical patients. *Haematologica* 2006;91:64–70.

5. Arcelus J, Caprini J, Motykie G *et al.* Matching risk with treatment strategies in deep vein thrombosis management. *Blood Coagulation and Fibrinolysis* 1999;10(Suppl 2): S37–43.

6. Bosson J, Labarere J. Determining indications for care common to competing guidelines by using classification tree analysis: application to the prevention of venous thromboembolism in medical inpatients. *Medical Decision Making* 2006;26:63–75.

7. Johnson M, Sherry K. How do palliative physicians manage venous thromboembolism? *Palliative Medicine* 1997;11(6):462–8.

8. Havig O. Deep venous thrombosis and pulmonary embolism: an autopsy study with multiple regression analysis of possible risk factors. *Acta Chirurgica Scandinavica* 1977;478(suppl):1–120.

9. Noble S, Nelson A, Turner C *et al.* Acceptability of low molecular weight heparin thromboprophylaxis for inpatients receiving palliative care: qualitative study. *British Medical Journal* 2006;332(7541):577–80.

10. Eddy DM. Variations in physician practice: the role of uncertainty. In: Dowie J, Elstein A, editors. *Professional judgement. A reader in clinical decision making.* Cambridge UK: Cambridge University Press; 1988. p. 45–59.

11. Chapman G, Sonnenberg F. Introduction. In: Chapman G, Sonnenberg F, editors. *Decision making in healthcare. Theory, Psychology and Applications.* Cambridge UK: Cambridge University Press; 2000. p. 3–19.

12. Sox H, Blatt M, Higgins M *et al. Medical Decision Making.* Boston: Butterworth-Heinemann; 1988.

13. Eraker S, Politser P. How decisions are reached. Physician and patient. In: Dowie J, Elstein A, editors. *Professional judgment. A reader in clinical decision making.* Cambridge UK: Cambridge University Press; 1988.

14. Tversky A, Kahneman D. Judgment under uncertainty: heuristics and biases. *Science* 1974;185:1124–31.

15. Chapman G, Elstein A. Cognitive processes and biases in medical decision making. In: Chapman G, Sonnenberg F, editors. *Decision making in healthcare. Theory, Psychology and Applications.* Cambridge UK: Cambridge University Press; 2000. p. 183–210.

16. Tversky A, Kahneman D. The framing of decisons and the psychology of choice. *Science* 1981;211:453–8.

17. Tversky A, Kahneman D. Rational choice and the framing of decisions. In: Bell D, Raiffa H, Tversky A, editors. *Decision making. Descriptive, normative and prescriptive interactions.* Cambridge UK: Cambridge University Press; 1988. p. 167–92.

18. Sackett D, Straus S, Richardson WS *et al. Evidence-based medicine. How to practice and teach EBM.* 2nd ed. Edinburgh: Churchill Livingstone; 2000.

19. Elwyn G, Edwards A, Eccles M *et al.* Decision analysis in patient care. *Lancet* 2001;358(2001 Aug 18):571–4.

20. Sarasin FP. Decision analysis and its application in clinical medicine. *European Journal of Obstetrics and Gynecology and Reproductive Biology* 2001;2001(94):172–9.

21. Tavakoli M, Davies HTO, Thomson R. Aiding clinical decisions with decision analysis. *Hospital Medicine* 1999;60(6):444–7.

22. Tavakoli M, Davies HTO, Thomson R. Decision analysis in evidence-based decision making. *Journal of Evaluation in Clinical Practice* 2000;6(2):111–20.

23. Thornton JG, Lilford RJ, Johnson N. Decision analysis in medicine. *British Medical Journal* 1992;304:1099–103.

24. Sarasin F, Eckman M. Management and prevention of thromboemoblic events in patients with cancer related hypercoagulable states: a risky business. *Journal of General Internal Medicine* 1993;8:476–86.

25. Thomson R, Parkin D, Eccles M *et al.* Decision analysis and guidelines for anticoagulant therapy to prevent stroke in patients with atrial fibrillation. *Lancet* 2000;355:956–62.

26. Robinson A, Thomson RG. The potential use of decision analysis to support shared decision making in the face of uncertainty: the example of atrial fibrillation and warfarin anticoagulation. *Quality in Health Care* 2000;9:238–44.

27. Protheroe J, Fahey T, Montgomery AA *et al.* The impact of patients' preferences on the treatment of atrial fibrillation: observational study of patient based decision analysis. *British Medical Journal* 2000;320:1380–4.

28. Man-Son-Hing M, Gage B, Montgomery AA *et al.* Preference-based antithrombotic therapy in atrial fibrillation: implications for clinical decision making. *Medical Decision Making* 2005;25:548–59.

29. Thomson RG, Eccles M, Steen I *et al.* A patient decision aid to support shared decision-making on anti-thrombotic treatment of patients with atrial fibrillation: randomised controlled trial. *Quality and Safety in Health Care* 2007;16:216–23.

30. Richardson WS, Detsky AS. Users' Guides to the medical literature VII How to use a clinical decision analysis B. What are the results and will they help me in caring for my patients? *The Journal of the American Medical Association* 1995;273(20):1610–3.

31. Hunink M, Glasziou P, Siegel J *et al. Decision making in health and medicine. Integrating evidence and values.* Cambridge UK: Cambridge University Press; 2001.

32. Chan A, Woodruff R. Complications and failure of anticoagulation therapy in the treatment of venous thromboembolism in patients with disseminated malignancy. *Australian and New Zealand Journal of Medicine* 1992;22:119–22.

33. Lee A, Levine M, Baker R *et al.* Low molecular weight heparin versus coumarin for the prevention of recurrent venous thromboembolism in patients with cancer. *The New England Journal of Medicine* 2003;349:146–53.

34. Hull R, Pineo G, Brant R *et al.* Long-term low molecular weight heparin versus usual care in proximal-vein thrombosis patients with cancer. *American Journal of Medicine* 2006;119:1062–72.

35. Kolachalam R, Julian T. Clinical presentation of thrombosed Greenfield filters. *Vascular Surgery* 1990;24:666–70.

Chapter 9

Venous thromboembolism in non-malignant disease

Anna Spathis and Sara Booth

Introduction

Many more people die from non-malignant disease than from cancer. In the developed world, approximately half of all deaths result from chronic non-malignant disease, whereas one-quarter is caused by cancer.[1,2] Palliative-care services, however, care for a disproportionate number of patients with malignant disease. This may reflect the fact that palliative care initially developed in the 1960s in response to the needs of terminally ill cancer patients. Less than 10 per cent of patients seen by specialist palliative-care teams in the UK have non-malignant disease.[3]

Over the last decade, there has been increasing recognition that patients with non-malignant disease have extensive palliative-care needs that are at least as great as those of patients with cancer.[4] Incurable chronic diseases such as heart failure (HF), chronic obstructive pulmonary disease (COPD), and cerebrovascular accident (CVA) or stroke can lead to a heavy symptom burden, emotional distress, and social isolation. There is evidence, for example, that patients with COPD have a quality of life that is as poor and, indeed, may be worse than that of patients with lung cancer.[5,6] Furthermore, the disease trajectories of non-cancer diagnoses typically show a prolonged functional decline, with worse performance status over a longer time than is usual in many types of cancer (Fig. 9.1).[7,8]

Venous thromboembolism (VTE) contributes significantly to the morbidity, and indeed mortality, of advanced non-malignant disease. Although cancer is undoubtedly a major risk factor for the development of thrombosis, VTE is just as prevalent in those with non-malignant conditions. Studies screening stroke patients show, for example, the incidence of asymptomatic deep vein thrombosis (DVT) to be in the range of 30–80 per cent without thromboprophylaxis.[9] Given that the majority of patients with advanced, incurable disease do not have cancer, VTE in non-malignant disease is clearly a topic of great importance.

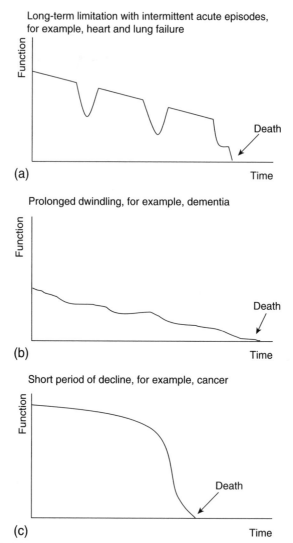

Fig. 9.1 Typical disease trajectories for progressive chronic illness. Reproduced with permission from British Medical Journal Publishing Group Ltd. From Murray SA, Kendall M, Boyd K. Illness trajectories and palliative care. *British Medical Journal* 2005; 330:1007–11.

This chapter provides an overview of existing evidence in relation to the management of VTE in noncancer diagnoses, and then attempts to apply this evidence to a palliative-care population with advanced, incurable disease. For palliative-care specialists with experience in caring for cancer patients, the aim is to increase awareness of issues relating to the management of VTE in non-malignant disease. For the many nonpalliative-care health professionals involved in the end-of-life care of those without cancer, the intention is to present current evidence from a palliative-care perspective, with its inherent focus on optimizing quality of life.

Prevalence

The epidemiology of VTE in advanced disease is described in detail in Chapter 2. A summary of data relevant to non-malignant disease is given here. The majority of research examining VTE in medical patients is conducted in the acute hospital setting. Although amongst hospital inpatients VTE is most often considered to be associated with recent surgery, 50–70 per cent of symptomatic thromboembolic events and 70–80 per cent of fatal pulmonary emboli (PEs) occur in nonsurgical patients.[10]

Unselected general medical inpatients are at a low to moderate risk of VTE when not receiving prophylaxis (Table 9.1). In a study of 234 consecutive medical admissions, excluding those with clinical suspicion of VTE and those on anticoagulants, the prevalence of asymptomatic DVT detected by venous compression ultrasonography was 5 per cent, increasing to 18 per cent amongst patients over 80 years of age.[11] Several large trials assessing the benefit of thromboprophylaxis have recruited higher-risk patients with congestive heart failure, acute or chronic respiratory illness, and infectious or inflammatory disease. DVT was found in 10–15 per cent of patients taking placebo, of which approximately one-third were proximal.[12–14]

Table 9.1 Levels of VTE risk in hospitalized medical patients without prophylaxis.[15]

Risk level	Risk DVT (per cent)	Risk PDVT* (per cent)	Risk fatal PE (per cent)	Patient groups
Low	<10	<1	0.01	Minor medical illness
Moderate	10–40	1–10	0.1–1	Major medical illness: heart or lung disease, inflammatory bowel disease, cancer. Minor medical illness in patients with previous VTE or thrombophilia
High	40–80	10–30	1–10	Major medical illness in patients with previous VTE or thrombophilia. Stroke with lower limb paralysis

*PDVT: proximal DVT

Several studies have assessed prevalence of VTE in individual advanced non-malignant diseases. A wide range of values are reported because of considerable heterogeneity in study populations and diagnostic methods.

HF

The majority of thromboembolic events in HF are arterial, and few studies have examined VTE rates in isolation.[16] The incidence of VTE amongst patients with HF (NYHA class III and IV) in the MEDENOX study was 14.6 per cent between days 1 and 14. In patients with the most severe HF (NYHA class IV), the incidence was 21.7 per cent. All study patients were screened for VTE with bilateral venography. Prevalence could not be calculated as patients with known VTE were excluded. These values are consistent with findings from autopsy studies, which reveal prevalence rates of 9–32 per cent.[17,18]

Several other studies have generated prevalence rates that are likely to be underestimates. Amongst 198 consecutive patients with severe decompensated HF, 18 (9 per cent) were found to have PE, despite 12 of these 18 patients using thromboprophylaxis.[19] Investigation for VTE was triggered by clinical suspicion, and asymptomatic VTE would have been missed. In a large survey of hospital discharge data, only 1.0 per cent and 0.7 per cent of patients with HF were diagnosed with DVT and PE respectively.[20] Data from death certificates have suggested that approximately 3 per cent of those with HF die from PE.[20] There is evidence, however, that death certificate diagnoses for PE are inaccurate, with a sensitivity for detection of PE of less than 30 per cent.[21,22]

COPD

In a study screening a population of 196 patients with COPD admitted to an intensive care unit, 10.7 per cent of patients were found to have DVT, and 86 per cent of these were asymptomatic.[23] This study will have underestimated the true prevalence as it excluded patients with cancer, HF, or previous VTE, and because ultrasound was used as the screening tool. In three other studies that screened patients using ultrasound, venography, and autologous platelet labelling with indium-111 (a method with poor specificity), DVT rates were 13.3, 28, and 45 per cent respectively.[24–26]

Two recent prospective studies have evaluated the prevalence of PE in consecutive patients admitted with a COPD exacerbation of unknown origin using spiral CT and ultrasonography. Rutschmann *et al.* found prevalence rates of 3 per cent whereas Tillie-Leblonde *et al.* found a much higher rate of 25 per cent.[27,28] This disparity reflects study population heterogeneity. Patients in the latter study were less well and were more likely to have additional risk factors such as cancer. Furthermore, patients were excluded with even a suggestion of chest infection, unlike the former study where only proven infection led to exclusion. In a large study conducted on 215 stable COPD patients on long-term oxygen therapy, PE appears to account for approximately 10 per cent of deaths.[29]

Stroke

Studies screening patients with acute hemiplegic stroke using I^{125}-fibrinogen scintigraphy or ultrasound have shown VTE rates of 20–80 per cent in the absence of thromboprophylaxis.[30] The majority of DVTs affect the paretic limb and are asymptomatic. A recent study that screened patients with direct magnetic resonance imaging of thrombus found prevalence values for all VTE, proximal DVT, and PE of 40, 18, and 12 per cent, respectively, increasing to 63, 30, and 20 per cent in those with most severe stroke (Barthel index 9 or less).[31] Recognized clinical DVT and PE occurred in only 1 and 3 per cent of patients, respectively. All patients were receiving standard thromboprophylaxis with aspirin and graded compression stockings (GCS). In one small study in patients with haemorrhagic stroke and no thromboprophylaxis, there was evidence of PE in 39 per cent using prospective screening with ventilation-perfusion (V/Q) scintigraphy.[32] Most DVTs develop in the first week after stroke, and the majority of fatal PE occur between the second and fourth weeks after stroke.[31,33]

Other advanced disease

Several other advanced diseases have been reported as being associated with an increased risk of VTE. In renal failure, for example, a review of autopsies has reported the prevalence of PE to be 12.5 per cent in chronic haemodialysis patients, and 22 per cent in nondialysis patients.[34] An increased annual DVT incidence of 2.7–3.0 per cent (compared to 1.3 per cent in all hospitalized patients) has been shown in patients with multiple sclerosis.[35,36]

Risk factors

Risk stratification in VTE is of great importance, as it is a condition where thromboprophylaxis can be targeted at higher risk patients. There has been extensive evaluation of precise risk factors in surgical patients. However, in medical patients—a heterogeneous group—few studies have examined this issue (Table 9.2).

The Sirius study was a large case-control study comparing risk factors in 636 outpatients with objectively confirmed DVT with 636 controls.[37] In a subgroup analysis of the 75 per cent of the study population that were medical patients, relevant risk factors in descending order of importance were: history of

Table 9.2 Risk factors for VTE in medical patients.[10,37,38,41]

Disease factors	Patient factors
HF (NYHA III and IV)*	History of VTE*
Acute infection*	Advanced age*
Cancer*	Immobility*
COPD exacerbation	Obesity*
Stroke with lower limb paresis	Venous insufficiency*
Renal failure	Dehydration
Inflammatory bowel disease	Smoking
Nephrotic syndrome	Hormone replacement therapy
Connective tissue disease	Central venous catheterization
Diabetes mellitus	Permanent pacemaker
Paroxysmal nocturnal haemaglobinuria	Hyperhomocysteinemia
	Inherited thrombophilia

* Major independent risk factors for VTE in advanced disease

VTE (odds ratio (OR) 15.6), deterioration in general condition (OR 5.75), immobility (OR 5.61), venous insufficiency (OR 4.45), chronic HF (OR 2.93), obesity (OR 2.39), long-distance travel (OR 2.35), and infectious disease (OR 1.95). Other factors, that tended towards but did not reach statistical significance, were cancer, inflammatory bowel disease, and rheumatological disease.

The MEDENOX study was conducted in 1102 medical inpatients to determine the efficacy of enoxaparin in preventing VTE.[14] This study is of particular interest as many patients had advanced chronic disease; approximately one-third had congestive cardiac failure (NYHA class III or IV), and half had chronic respiratory failure. Previous VTE (2.06), acute infectious disease (OR 1.74), cancer (OR 1.62), and age older than 75 years (OR 1.03) were found by multiple logistic regression analysis to be independent risk factors for VTE.[38] There is consistent evidence from these and other studies that risk factors are cumulative in their effect, with increasing VTE events as the number of risk factors increases.[37–40]

HF

One retrospective case-control study has identified congestive HF as an independent risk factor for VTE.[41] The study population was predominantly medical, with only 4 per cent of patients having had recent surgery. Logistic regression analysis identified three other strong independent risk factors for VTE in medical patients: prior VTE, recent surgery, and obesity. Importantly, risk of VTE increased significantly with declining left ventricular ejection fraction (LVEF). Patients with an LVEF of less than 20 per cent had a very high risk of VTE, with an OR of 38.3 when compared to study patients without available LVEF measurement.

Amongst patients with HF, only one study has examined factors that increase risk of VTE. In a study population with severe, decompensated HF, Darze *et al.* found three strong and independent risk factors for PE: cancer, right ventricular abnormality, and previous VTE.[19]

COPD

There is no clear evidence that COPD is an independent risk factor for VTE. Evidence for increased VTE prevalence in COPD comes largely from studies in patients with exacerbations of COPD. It appears to be a risk factor due to its close association with established risk factors, such as infection, advanced age, immobility, right ventricular failure, and venous stasis.[42] Akgun *et al.* found that VTE occurred more commonly in COPD patients with worse dyspnoea, lower performance status, and a long-distance travel history within the last two weeks, all of which involve reduced mobility.[24]

It is likely that smoking is another associated risk factor that contributes to the prevalence of VTE in COPD. There is some evidence from large studies that smoking is an independent risk factor for VTE events.[43,44] However, this is a controversial issue, as other studies have failed to find any association between smoking and VTE.[45]

Stroke

Although patients with CVA and lower limb paresis have one of the highest risks of VTE amongst medical patients, the existence of a CVA is not in itself an independent risk factor for VTE. Again, as with COPD, it is the association of CVA with other strong risk factors that leads to the high prevalence of VTE in these patients. The role of immobility as the primary risk factor is high-lighted by the consistently higher rates in the paretic limb.[31,46] Additional associated risk factors include dehydration, due to dysphagia and poor oral intake, and advanced age.[47] Amongst patients with CVA, the risk of VTE has been shown to be higher with increasing stroke severity, haemorrhagic stroke, previous VTE, postphlebitic syndrome, disseminated malignancy, and congestive heart failure.[31,47–49]

Other advanced disease

Other than HF, there is no evidence that any other non-malignant conditions are independent risk factors for VTE. It is likely that the risk of VTE increases in such conditions because of established risk factors including immobility, increasing age, and dehydration.[35] Evidence from a Spanish registry of over 10,000 consecutive patients with VTE shows that risk factors for fatal PE in patients with renal failure include creatinine clearance (CrCl) less than 30, immobility, and cancer.[50] There is inconsistent data as to whether or not dialysis itself is a risk factor.[34,51] There is some evidence from a series of case reports that venous thrombosis may occur as a complication of venous haemodialysis access.[52]

In multiple sclerosis, reduced mobility is likely to be the major risk factor.[36] High-dose methylprednisolone may influence coagulation and appears to be associated with an increased risk of cerebral venous thrombosis. Although unproven, it may be a risk factor for DVT and PE in such patients.[53,54]

Pathogenesis

In 1884, Virchow proposed that thrombosis was the consequence of at least three factors: stasis of blood flow, hypercoagulability of blood, and vascular endothelial damage. All risk factors for VTE reflect these three underlying pathophysiological processes.[40]

HF

Occurrence of thrombosis in HF is intuitively likely because stasis or deceleration of blood flow is caused by poor cardiac contractility. This is, however, not the only mechanism. HF also causes ischaemic vascular endothelial damage and confers a state of hypercoagulability.

Peripheral tissue hypoxia occurs because of poor perfusion caused by inadequate cardiac function. Activation of the sympathetic and renin-aldosterone systems contribute to tissue hypoxia by causing peripheral vasoconstriction. Ischaemic endothelium releases the adhesion molecule P-selectin, which binds leukocytes. These, in turn, release procoagulant tissue factor, which can initiate the coagulation cascade.[55,56] Furthermore, tissue hypoxia stimulates the production of proinflammatory cytokines, including tumour necrosis factor-α, interleukin-1β, and interleukin-6, which induce further tissue factor formation, accelerate coagulation reactions, and inhibit the endogenous fibrinolytic system.[57–59]

This prothrombotic state in HF can be viewed as a maladaptive inflammatory response.[60] As discussed above, it is known that the risk of VTE increases with declining ejection fraction, and there is evidence that the levels of some of these biochemical markers increase as LVEF falls.[61] Drugs that inhibit the renin-aldosterone system have been shown to improve levels of procoagulant and inflammatory factors, lessening the prothrombotic state.[60]

COPD

COPD can lead to right ventricular dysfunction, triggering venous stasis, endothelial damage, and an inflammatory response as described above. In addition, the condition frequently causes reduced mobility due to disabling dyspnoea. Immobility, one of the most consistently strong risk factors for VTE in all patient groups, leads to thrombosis by causing venous stasis, and lower limb haemoconcentration.[10,62]

VTE events are clearly associated with COPD exacerbations, which are usually infective in origin. The mechanism by which infection, an independent risk factor for VTE in medical patients, causes thrombosis has not been clearly established. However, it is likely to involve interaction between the inflammatory and coagulation pathways described above.

There is some evidence that active smoking may be a contributor to the risk of VTE, and several mechanisms have been proposed.[43,63] Chronic smokers exhibit a mild, but sustained, acute-phase response, characterized by increased plasma concentrations of procoagulant tissue factor and inflammatory cytokines.[64,65] Factor VIII covalently cross-links and stabilizes fibrin clots, and levels have been found to be elevated in smokers.[63] Effective fibrinolysis requires rapid tissue plasminogen activator (tPA) release from endothelium. Smokers have been found to have impaired capacity for tPA release.[66]

Stroke

The predominant mechanism for VTE in CVA is venous stasis, caused primarily by immobility from lower limb paralysis. Although it seems intuitively probable that dehydration, an established risk factor in CVA, could lead to VTE by causing haemoconcentration and increased coagulation, the evidence to support this is unclear. There is an increased risk of thrombosis in myeloproliferative disorders that cause erythrocytosis, such as polycythaemia rubra vera. Other than this, there is, however, little evidence that a raised haematocrit increases coagulation, although haemoconcentration may increase net thrombus volume.[68–70] It may be that dehydration acts as a risk factor for CVA by its correlation with disease severity.

Other advanced disease

In renal failure, an antithrombotic tendency due to platelet abnormalities caused by uraemia is well recognized. However, there is also evidence of hypercoagulability and endothelial damage occurring, which may contribute to the significantly increased VTE risk. Levels of proinflammatory cytokines and procoagulant factors have been consistently shown to be raised in renal failure, suggesting mechanisms similar to those believed to occur in HF. In addition, biochemical abnormalities may occur as a consequence of dialysis. Both hyper-homocysteinaemia, a well-established risk factor for thrombosis, and protein C deficiency have been shown to occur in patients on long-term dialysis.[70]

Consequences of VTE

The majority of DVTs originate in the calf. Distal DVTs seldom embolize, are rarely symptomatic and only 10–20 per cent progress to proximal DVTs.[71] The consequences of an untreated distal DVT are therefore relatively minor. 10–30 per cent of DVTs are proximal.[12,14,72] These are, by contrast, usually symptomatic, and approximately 50 per cent of patients with untreated proximal DVT will develop symptomatic PE within three months.[73] One-quarter of symptomatic PE are fatal.[74] Medical patients have a greater mortality following VTE than surgical patients.[75] Furthermore, there is consistent evidence that those with advanced disease, including HF, COPD, CVA, and renal failure, have poorer outcomes than general medical patients.[24,76,77] This is unsurprising given that such patients have a poor cardiopulmonary reserve, rendering them less likely to tolerate an embolic event.

Resolution of proximal DVT in anticoagulated patients is slow. After 6 months treatment, over 50 per cent of patients have residual thrombus, and in 5–10 per cent there is extension of thrombus despite treatment.[78] The risk of recurrent VTE after stopping anticoagulant therapy is approximately 20 per cent after 2 years averaged across all patient groups, but the risk depends largely on whether the initial thrombus was associated with a transient or per-manent risk factor.[73,79] Although patients with non-malignant disease typically experience a longer period of decline than patients with advanced cancer, and therefore may be considered at higher risk of recurrent VTE, this may be offset by the fact that risk factors are more likely to be transient, as discussed later in this chapter.

The post-thrombotic syndrome (PTS) is a prevalent consequence of VTE that causes significant morbidity. It is largely caused by venous hypertension secondary to residual thrombus and venous valve damage. Patients complain of pain, heaviness, swelling, and itching of the leg, typically aggravated by standing. Skin changes can occur that include varicose eczema, hyperpigmen-tation, and in severe cases, lipodermatosclerosis and ulceration.

Two recent prospective studies have assessed the incidence of PTS in patients with DVT who were anticoagulated for 3 months. Brandjes et al. found that 60 per cent of patients developed PTS within 2 years, and 24 per cent had severe PTS.[80] Prandoni et al. found rather lower values of approximately 25 and 6 per cent, respectively at 2 years, and an incidence of 18 per cent at

1 year.[81] The disparity in outcomes may reflect the different scoring systems used to define the syndrome. Risk factors for PTS development are increasing age and recurrent VTE.[82] Established PTS cannot be easily treated, although there is some evidence that intractable symptoms can be reduced with long-term use of graduated compression stockings or an intermittent extremity compression pump.[80,82,83]

PTS has a significantly negative impact on disease-specific quality of life.[84] It is relatively neglected syndrome and its importance has not been appreciated in palliative-care literature to date.[85] This may be because it is erroneously perceived to be a long-term consequence of VTE.[86] However, there is good evidence that the vast majority of cases of PTS become apparent within 2 years following of DVT.[79,80] As many patients, particularly those with non-malignant disease, live with advanced incurable disease for longer than this, PTS is an important syndrome that should have a higher profile.

As well as many advanced non-malignant conditions increasing the risk of VTE, venous thrombosis can itself cause incurable and serious medical disease. Chronic embolic pulmonary hypertension is associated with significant morbidity and mortality. Although considered to be rare in the past, it has recently been shown to occur in approximately 4 per cent of patients, within the 2 years after a first symptomatic PE event.[87]

Venous thromboses do not just embolize to the lung. In patients with a patent foramen ovale (PFO), thrombus may cross to the arterial circulation and cause stroke. The cause of ischaemic stroke is never found in approximately 40 per cent of patients, and amongst those with cryptogenic stroke, the prevalence of PFO is 44–66 per cent. Embolism through a PFO is believed to be the mechanism in an unknown but potentially significant proportion of patients with cryptogenic stroke.[88,89]

Diagnosis

In patients with advanced incurable disease, the aim of medical care is to improve quality of life. It is, therefore, particularly important to diagnose conditions, such as VTE, that have a negative impact on quality of life and are relatively easily treatable. Accurate diagnosis of VTE can be challenging since as few as one-tenth of VTE events are associated with symptoms.[13] Furthermore, in many advanced conditions, particularly HF and COPD, clinical features of the disease may mask or mimic VTE. In essence, diagnosis is most difficult in those patients least able to tolerate a VTE event.[76]

The diagnosis of VTE in advanced disease is covered extensively in Chapter 4 and the discussion is relevant to non-malignant as well as malignant disease. The main issue specific to non-malignant disease is the impact of concurrent pathology on the validity of clinical features and imaging. Two common and challenging clinical scenarios are the diagnosis of PE in patients with exacerbation of COPD, and differentiation between PE and pneumonia in those with CVA.

The symptoms and signs of PE resemble an exacerbation of COPD so closely, it is often impossible to distinguish them by clinical assessment alone. This can lead to significant underdiagnosis.[90] In the PIOPED study, out of 108 patients with COPD suspected of having a PE, the clinical features of those who did have confirmed PE did not differ significantly from those without.[91] Furthermore, the diagnostic value of V/Q scintigraphy is decreased in patients with COPD, as structural alterations in the pulmonary vasculature may result in changes in ventilation-perfusion relationships.[92,93] More than double the number of V/Q scan results are nondiagnostic in COPD patients compared to those without COPD, with indeterminate scan rates of 40–60 per cent.[91,94]

However, it should not be forgotten that the accurate diagnosis of PE can be problematic even in those without COPD. Diagnosis frequently requires information from multiple tools, including clinical probability assessment, noninvasive screening such as D-dimer assay, and radiological investigations such as V/Q scanning and spiral computed tomographic angiography (SCTA).[95] In the ANTELOPE study, the presence of COPD did not significantly change the accuracy and performance of any of these methods, other than an increased proportion of nondiagnostic V/Q scans.[94] The authors conclude that, although V/Q scintigraphy is less cost-effective in the presence of COPD, because of its unchanged sensitivity and specificity, it remains a useful tool in COPD patients.

A number of factors make diagnosis of PE more difficult in CVA patients. Patients may not complain of symptoms because of dysphasia or cognitive impairment.[96] Furthermore, pneumonia is very common after CVA, and can be notoriously hard to differentiate from PE.[97] In a case series in which 21 patients were found to have both pneumonia and major PE, the latter diagnosis was not suspected in a single case antemortem.[98] They share considerable overlap in their clinical features; even fever and leukocytosis are common in PE.[99] In addition, the conditions commonly coexist, each predisposing a patient to the other.

There has been little research examining this topic, evaluating the discriminatory value of clinical factors. In the absence of such data, clinicians should increase their index of suspicion for PE in patients with apparent pneumonia. There may be value in looking, for example, for a degree of hypoxia incommensurate with the extent of consolidation or electrocardiogram changes suggestive of PE. Infection tends to increase D-dimer levels, but the sensitivity of the test remains high. Therefore, in both infective exacerbations of COPD and CVA with pneumonia, a low D-dimer level remains a useful tool for excluding PE. Spiral CT is likely to be a more useful initial investigation than V/Q scintigraphy in the presence of consolidation.[97]

Management

Treatment and secondary prevention

In advanced non-malignant disease, issues of drug choice, safety, and duration of administration are much the same as in advanced cancer and, having already been covered in detail in Chapters 5 and 6, will only be considered briefly here. As in cancer, low molecular weight heparins (LMWHs) are most likely to be used for initiation of treatment, in place of unfractionated heparin (UFH). Although warfarin is conventionally used for maintenance of anticoagulation, LMWHs have a number of advantages in advanced disease, in that they do not require laboratory monitoring and have a more uniform anticoagulant effect compared to warfarin—due to less influence from diet—nutritional status and drug interactions.[100]

The major risk of anticoagulation is bleeding, the incidence of which increases significantly with reduced performance status, concurrent use of antiplatelet drugs, comorbid illness, advanced age, and higher anticoagulant drug doses.[101–104] Concerns about bleeding on anticoagulants are just as pertinent in patients with non-malignant disease as in patients with cancer. Those with advanced non-malignant disease tend to experience a lower performance status for longer than those with advanced cancer. Furthermore, many more patients with HF and stroke are likely to be taking aspirin for secondary prevention of vascular disease. Comorbid illnesses associated with increased bleeding risk include ischaemic stroke,[102,105–108] congestive HF[109–111] and renal failure.[50,102,109,112] Even in these conditions, however, there is consistent evidence that the balance of risks lies in favour of full-dose anticoagulation, because of the significant morbidity and mortality associated with untreated VTE.[50,108] Anticoagulation is clearly contraindicated following haemorrhagic stroke.

Patients who have an irreversible, strong risk factor, such as cancer, should mostly be anticoagulated indefinitely in order to prevent recurrent VTE. However, for patients with reversible risk factors, the recommendation is that they should be anticoagulated for 3 months only.[113–115] Unlike cancer, in advanced non-malignant disease the condition itself appears not to be an independent risk factor (with the exception of HF), and there is an increased likelihood that the risk factors may be reversible. Following a stroke with limb paresis, for example, the tendency is towards neurological improvement and a degree of recovery of function. This means that the main risk factor in such patients, immobility, may no longer present. Most DVTs occur in the first week after stroke, and the vast majority within the first month. In some similar patients, therefore, it could be reasonable to stop anticoagulation after just 3 months.[113] In COPD, once an infective exacerbation has resolved, two of the main risk factors—infection and immobility due to dyspnoea—may have also improved. Again, indefinite anticoagulation may be unnecessary. In severe HF, however, the situation is more analogous to cancer, in that the disease itself—the main risk factor—cannot be reversed. Long-term anticoagulation for secondary prevention may therefore be appropriate.

Primary prevention

Given the high prevalence of VTE, the considerable adverse consequences that are hard to treat, such as PE and PTS, and the poor outcomes in those with advanced non-malignant disease, the rationale for primary prevention is strong. Thromboprophylaxis in medical patients is, however, a contentious issue and has been the subject of extensive research and heated debate in recent years.[10,75,116,117] This topic has been covered in some detail in Chapter 7, and is therefore only summarized here, with particular reference to non-malignant disease.

Routine use of thromboprophylaxis is firmly established in surgical patients, as the risk for VTE can be determined by the type of surgery and generally only short-term prophylaxis is required.[118] The cost-effectiveness in surgical patients has been proven beyond doubt.[10] Medical patients, however, form a more heterogeneous population with less easily quantifiable risk. Furthermore, the larger numbers of patients involved and the potentially longer requirement for prophylaxis have lead to concerns about possible harms of treatment and the lack of evidence for cost-effectiveness.[119]

Dentali *et al.* have recently conducted a meta-analysis of nine randomized controlled trials comparing anticoagulant prophylaxis with no treatment in hospitalized medical patients (Table 9.3).[119] Study patients were considered to be of moderate risk and were predominantly patients with HF (NYHA III-IV), acute, or chronic respiratory disease, and infectious or rheumatological disease. Only one study involved patients entirely with advanced disease, an evaluation of nadroparin in ventilated patients with acute, decompensated COPD.[25] All trials involved short-term use of anticoagulants for generally less than 14 days.

Table 9.3 Studies evaluating thromboprophylaxis in medical patients.[119]

Study	Indication for prophylaxis	Drug regimen	RR symptomatic DVT (95 per cent CI)	RR PE (95 per cent CI)
Belch[120]	HF, chest infection	UH, 5,000 U three times daily	—	0.20 (0.01–4.06)
Dahan[121]	Congestive HF (NYHA III-IV), acute or respiratory infectious disease	Enoxaparin, 60 mg once daily	—	0.33 (0.03–3.14)
Gärdlund[122]	Infectious disease	UH, 5,000 U twice daily	—	0.26 (0.07–0.91)
Samama[14]	Congestive HF (NYHA III-IV), acute or chronic respiratory disease, acute infectious or rheumatologic disease	Enoxaparin, 40 mg once daily	0.49 (0.05–5.43)	0.14 (0.01–2.73)
Fraisse[25]	Acute decompensated COPD with mechanical ventilation	Nadroparin, 3,800–5,700 U once daily	—	—
Leizorovicz[12]	Congestive HF (NYHA III-IV), acute or chronic respiratory disease, infectious and rheumatologic disease	Dalteparin, 5,000 U once daily	0.45 (0.16–1.29)	1.24 (0.33–4.60)
Mahé[123]	Congestive HF (NYHA III-IV), acute or respiratory disease, nonpulmonary sepsis, cancer	Nadroparin, 7,500 U once daily	—	0.59 (0.27–1.29)
Lederle[124]	Hospitalisation in general medical unit	Enoxaparin, 4,000 U once daily	0.50 (0.15–1.62)	0.33 (0.04–3.17)
Cohen[13]	Congestive HF (NYHA III-IV), acute respiratory, infectious or inflammatory disease	Fondaparinux, 2.5 mg once daily	—	0.09 (0.00–1.60)

The principle findings were that thromboprophylaxis led to a significant reduction in PE by more than 50 per cent (relative risk, RR 0.43, 95 per cent confidence intervals (CI), 0.26–0.71) and fatal PE (RR 0.38, CI 0.21–0.69), a non-significant reduction in symptomatic DVT (RR 0.47, CI 0.22–1.00) and a non-significant increase in major bleeding (RR 1.32, CI 0.73–2.37). The number needed to treat (NNT) to avoid one PE was 345. Anticoagulant use had no effect on all-cause mortality. In the study involving patients with advanced COPD, the risk of asymptomatic DVT was reduced by approximately 45 per cent.[25] The researchers concluded that the use of thromboprophylaxis should be limited to higher risk patients such as those with congestive HF, respiratory disease, active cancer, previous VTE, sepsis, and acute inflammatory disease. This view is consistent with that of the seventh American College of Chest Physicians (ACCP) conference guideline on thromboprophylaxis, which recommends that prophylactic anticoagulation should be given to 'acutely ill medical patients who have admitted to hospital with congestive heart failure or severe respiratory disease, or who are confined to bed and have one or more additional risk factors, including active cancer, previous VTE, sepsis, acute neurological disease, or inflammatory bowel disease.'[10]

Post-hoc subgroup analysis of a large study in the meta-analysis by Dentali et al., the MEDENOX trial, examined the effect of prophylactic LMWH on each disease group, and found significant reduction in VTE for all disease categories, including chronic HF (RR 0.25, CI 0.08–0.92) and chronic respiratory failure (RR 0.26, CI 0.10–0.69). A recent systematic review of studies in ischaemic stroke with limb paresis concluded that prophylactic anticoagulation prevented VTE with an NNT of 2–10. The benefits were lost when unselected stroke patients received prophylaxis.[30] Kelly et al. have calculated that for every 100 patients with stroke treated with low-dose LMWH, approximately 15 fatal PEs, 30 nonfatal clinical PEs, and 11 recurrent ischaemic strokes may be prevented, at a cost of six intracranial and six extracranial haemorrhages.[31]

There is increasing consensus in the literature that low-dose LMWHs are the anticoagulant of choice for thromboprophylaxis in medical patients.[125] A meta-analysis of nine studies comparing LMWH with UFH in acutely ill medical patients has found a nonsignificant trend in favour of LMWH in reduction of DVT (RR 0.83, CI 0.56–1.24 and of PE (RR 0.74, CI 0.29–1.80), and a marginal reduction in major bleeding (RR 0.48, CI 0.23–1.0).[126] A study comparing LMWH with UFH in patients with NYHA III or IV HF or severe respiratory disease found that LMWH had at least the same efficacy as UFH, with a superior safety profile.[127] In patients with stroke, prophylactic doses of LMWH appear to be more effective than UFH, adverse events being low with both drugs.[127] The NNT with LMWH to avoid one VTE is 13, whereas the number needed to harm as a result of clinically important bleeding is 173.[125] Low-dose LMWH is safer in stroke than high-dose LMWH and any dose of UFH.[129] LMWHs have been found to be more cost-effective than UFH in high-risk medical patients, lower total hospital costs outweighing increased drug costs.[130]

The ACCP thromboprophylaxis guideline recommends against use of aspirin alone as prophylaxis against VTE in any patient group.[10] The evidence in relation to aspirin use is inconsistent.[30,131] Data from two large meta-analyses and several other trials suggest that even low-dose aspirin does reduce VTE risk.[132–134] In other studies, mainly in surgical patients, there appears to be no benefit.[135,136] There is, however, consistent evidence that aspirin has inferior efficacy compared to other forms of thromboprophylaxis. In patients with stroke, for example, the NNT to prevent one VTE appears to be over 700.[10,30] Most patients with stroke and HF will be already taking low-dose aspirin for secondary prevention of vascular disease. Although there have, as yet, been no studies directly assessing the safety of low-dose aspirin combined with low-dose LMWH in patients at risk of bleeding complications, such as those with stroke, the consensus is that the combination is likely to be safe.[137]

Unlike in surgical patients where there is good evidence that graded compression stockings (GCS) reduce peri-operative VTE incidence,[138] there has just been one study evaluating their effectiveness in preventing VTE in medical patients.[139] This small, randomized study in patients with CVA found a trend towards VTE reduction that was not statistically significant. GCS are generally poorly tolerated, and there is evidence from patients with advanced cancer that they have a negative impact on quality of life.[140] Their use is, therefore, not recommended in medical patients, other than for use in patients in whom anticoagulation is contraindicated, such as following haemorrhagic CVA.[10,141,142] GCS cannot be used in patients with diabetic or other sensory neuropathy.

Despite the consensus that thromboprophylaxis should be given to high-risk medical patients, there is clear evidence for significant underutilization of thromboprophylaxis in this group.[75,143–145] Reasons for this may include a lack of awareness of the high prevalence of asymptomatic VTE in such patients, concern about bleeding risk, and uncertain cost-effectiveness. The lack of validated risk assessment model (RAM) in medical patients, to aid selection of those at higher risk, is also likely to be an important factor.[144,146–148] RAMs can involve assigning a score based on the presence of certain risk factors, and using the score to determine risk category and appropriate intervention. Some novel RAMs applicable to medical patients are in the process of being developed.[149–151]

Applying the evidence

Evidence based medicine forms the bedrock of modern medical care. One of its major limitations, however, is the difficulty in extrapolating evidence from studies to individual patients. To what extent can the evidence described above be applied to patients with advanced non-malignant disease?

Research issues

Very few of the studies evaluating VTE in non-malignant disease focus on patients with advanced disease. Almost all the studies described above involved hospitalized general medical patients, of whom many had acute disease, often infectious in origin. Fraisse *et al.* undertook the only study in patients entirely with advanced disease.[25] However, even this study population—patients ventilated following COPD decompensation—is not necessarily typical of those with advanced disease.

Although a significant proportion of patients in these studies did have incurable non-malignant disease, such as HF or COPD, it is not clear how advanced such diseases were in each study population. Research in vulnerable patients with very advanced disease is fraught with ethical and methodological concerns.[152,153] In practice, this means that the majority of studies exclude patients with the most advanced disease.

It is, therefore, likely that much of the data generated by these studies may not be applicable to a population with advanced non-malignant disease, receiving palliative care. There is consistent evidence that VTE risk increases with increasing disease severity and, therefore, many of the quoted prevalence rates in non-malignant disease may be underassessments.[24,41,49] Missed diagnoses are more likely in patients with advanced disease, as concurrent symptoms may mask symptoms of VTE. In addition, patients with more severe disease may have less cardio-respiratory reserve, and experience greater morbidity and mortality following VTE than a general medical population with less advanced disease. The risk of bleeding on anticoagulants will also be greater in those with advanced disease, both because HF, CVA, and renal failure are independent risk factors for increased bleeding, and because other risk factors, such as older age and reduced performance status will be more prevalent.

As well as these issues in relation to study population, the design of most existing studies further reduce their applicability to patients with more advanced disease. The most commonly used outcome measures assess rates of VTE events and survival. In patients with more advanced disease, the focus of care is on improving quality of life. Factors such as impact on symptom control, acceptability of treatments, and psychosocial issues become much more important than, for example, rates of asymptomatic DVT, and survival.

Most of the small amount of existing research that evaluate VTE from a quality of life perspective, have been undertaken by palliative care specialists.[140,154] As such, specialists tend to care mainly for patients with cancer diagnoses, the research naturally focuses on patients with malignant disease. Is research evidence gathered from advanced cancer patients applicable to those with advanced non-malignant disease?

As discussed before, advanced malignant and non-malignant diseases are not always comparable. Many more patients have advanced non-cancer diagnoses. Furthermore, the disease trajectories of those with non-malignant disease typically involve a less good level of function for a longer time than that experienced by cancer patients. Patients with organ failure, such as HF or COPD, are inherently less stable than cancer patients for much of their disease trajectory, and can experience a sudden and profound deterioration in conditions following even a minor insult.

These differences mean that extrapolation of evidence between the two populations is not necessarily reliable. The relative importance of management issues can vary between the two groups. For example, in patients with non-malignant disease, the longer trajectory means that secondary prevention, complications such as PTS, burdens of treatment, and cost-effectiveness issues become of even greater importance. Conversely, some of the problems discussed in other chapters in relation to cancer patients could be less of a concern. For example, the short, dramatic, and often reversible deteriorations in patients with organ failure mean that such patients are often hospitalized during such an event. Investigations are easier to perform in this context, and it is clearer when prophylaxis should be used. In addition, as patients with non-malignant disease tend to be cared for by non-palliative-care health professionals, there is less likely to be the cultural antipathy to the principles of prophylaxis that can occur in the palliative care context.[155]

Overall, therefore, the current evidence base in relation to patients with advanced non-malignant disease is inadequate. It is difficult to extrapolate evidence both from non-malignant populations with less advanced disease, and from cancer populations with advanced disease. There is an urgent need for research in patients with advanced non-malignant disease to address the large number of important and unanswered questions.

Management issues

The ACCP recommendations on antithrombotic and thrombolytic therapy describe two methods for making decisions in relation to thromboprophylaxis.

One approach is to make group-specific recommendations, managing all patients within each target group in the same way. The other is to consider the risk of VTE in each patient, based on an individual's risk factors. They support the former approach because of several reasons.[10] First, an individualized approach has not been subjected to rigorous research evaluation, and second, such an approach would be more logistically complex and more likely to be associated with suboptimal compliance. Therefore, the ACCP recommendations are all group-based.

This viewpoint is diametrically opposed to that of the patient-centred palliative care philosophy. Patients with advanced disease are a heterogeneous and poorly defined group, with diverse symptoms and psychosocial needs. Care must be individualized, addressing the issues concerning each patient, in order to achieve the aim of improving quality of life.

Therefore, although current evidence can be used as guidance, the key to the management of VTE in patients with advanced non-malignant disease is to undertake individual clinical assessments. Each patient should be evaluated separately, taking into account prognosis, personal, and disease-related risk factors, and the likely benefits and burdens of each intervention. Quality of life is paramount. Until the evidence base is stronger in this patient group, it is not possible, or indeed desirable, for institutions to develop protocols or policies to govern the management of VTE in the patients with advanced non-malignant disease.

As the majority of research in patients with non-malignant disease is not conducted in the highest risk patients with the most advanced disease, optimal management of VTE in such patients may differ from currently accepted guidance. For example, it has been proposed that in patients with paretic stroke, the risk of asymptomatic VTE is so high that there may be a role for screening such patients to look for undiagnosed VTE.[156] The choice of screening tool does, however, present some difficulties. Ultrasound is specific, but lacks sensitivity, whereas D-dimer levels, which increase in the acute phase of many illnesses including stroke, lack specificity.[156,157] A single D-dimer assay at day 9 poststroke has been shown to identify a subgroup with approximately 50 per cent prevalence of proximal DVT.[158] There is some evidence that screening in stroke with ultrasound can be cost-effective.[159]

Although aspirin is not advocated for thromboprophylaxis, in a small proportion of medical patients with advanced disease and a higher risk of bleeding, it may be the most appropriate choice of prophylaxis.[131] It does not require painful injections, can be easily used in the community, and is associated with a lower risk of bleeding than low-dose anticoagulation. Clearly, further research in patients with advanced disease is of vital importance to determine effective, tolerated, and cost-effective management options in this vulnerable population.

Practical guidance

- Patients with advanced non-malignant disease can have as high a risk of VTE as those with advanced cancer, and therefore a high index of suspicion for established DVT or for PE events should be maintained at all times.

- As with cancer patients, established VTE should be treated with full-dose LMWH. Warfarin may be unsafe in a significant proportion of patients, and long-term LMWH, either by self-injection or daily injection by a community nurse, may be used instead.

- When the main underlying risk factor is reversible and/or the risk of bleeding is significant, treatment should be maintained for 3 months. If the main risk factor is not reversible, indefinite anticoagulation should be considered.

- In all patients, an individual clinical assessment should be undertaken, evaluating the risk of VTE and discussing the likely benefits and burdens of thromboprophylaxis.

- High-risk patients, particularly those with HF or stroke with leg paresis, should be considered for thromboprophylaxis with low-dose LMWH during any period of acute deterioration, particularly if there is associated infection or reduction in mobility. Thromboprophylaxis will usually be required for no more than 2 weeks.

- Patients entering the terminal phase or those considered likely to die during an admission to hospital or specialist palliative-care unit are unlikely to benefit from thromboprophylaxis.

- Aspirin is less effective than LMWH for thromboprophylaxis. However, it is taken by a significant proportion of patients with non-malignant conditions as secondary prevention of vascular disease, and it may have a role in VTE prophylaxis in the few patients who cannot tolerate LMWH.

- Graduated compression stockings are rarely useful in this patient group as they have an adverse effect on quality of life. If tolerated, they can be used for thromboprophylaxis when anticoagulation is contra-indicated, such as in haemorrhagic stroke, and they may have a role in the treatment of post-thrombotic syndrome.

Conclusion

Many more people are suffering from advanced non-malignant disease than from cancer. The risk of VTE in medical patients with non-malignant disease is just as high as the risk in cancer patients. However, the evidence base underpinning the management of VTE in advanced non-cancer patients is inadequate, and evidence from acute medical patients with less advanced disease or from cancer patients with advanced disease cannot easily be extrapolated to this patient group. There is an urgent need for rigorous research to try to determine the prevalence, impact, and appropriate treatment of VTE in patients with advanced non-malignant disease. In the meantime, the cornerstone of management should be careful clinical assessment of individual patients to establish the potential benefits and burdens of investigation, treatment, and thromboprophylaxis.

Key points

- Patients with advanced non-malignant disease may be at as great a risk for VTE as cancer patients, experiencing VTE prevalence rates of 10–50 per cent.
- Amongst patients with advanced non-malignant disease, those with stroke-associated lower limb paresis have the highest risk.
- Heart failure is the only non-malignant disease believed to be an independent risk factor for VTE. In other conditions, the risk comes from multiple associated traditional risk factors.
- In advanced non-malignant disease, the two main mechanisms for thrombosis formation are immobility causing venous stasis and development of an inflammatory, prothrombotic state, particularly during periods of acute deterioration.
- PTS is a prevalent and neglected consequence of VTE that causes considerable morbidity, and is of particular concern in non-malignant disease with its potentially longer disease trajectory and lower performance status.
- Diagnosis of VTE in non-malignant disease can be challenging as the clinical features of the condition, such as dyspnoea in HF, COPD, or stroke with concurrent pneumonia, may mimic or obscure symptoms of PE.
- Many non-malignant conditions, including HF, stroke, and renal failure are associated with an increased risk of bleeding with anticoagulation.
- Compared to cancer patients, patients with non-malignant disease are less likely to need indefinite treatment for secondary prevention of VTE, as the risk factors are more often short-term or reversible.

◆ Individual clinical assessments are needed to determine the risk of VTE and the likely benefits and burdens of thromboprophylaxis. Low-dose LMWH can be an appropriate intervention in selected high-risk patients during inpatient admission.

◆ There is an urgent need for research specifically in patients with advanced non-malignant disease, as existing evidence from those with cancer or with less advanced disease cannot easily be extrapolated to this patient group.

References

1. DOH. Mortality statistics; cause, England and Wales. London: National Statistics; 2005.

2. Centers for Disease Control & Prevention. *The burden of chronic diseases and their risk factors*: National & State Perspectives 2004. http://www.cdc-gov/nccdphp/burdenbook 2004.(Accessed February 2004).

3. NCPC. *Minimum dataset report 2005/6*. London: National Council for Palliative Care; 2006.

4. Addington-Hall J. *Reaching out: specialist palliative care for adults with non-malignant disease*. London: National Council for Hospices and Specialist Palliative Care Services; 1998. Occasional Paper 14.

5. Edmonds P, Karlsen S, Khan S *et al*. A comparison of the palliative care needs of patients dying from chronic respiratory diseases and lung cancer. *Palliative Medicine* 2001;15(4):287–95.

6. Gore JM, Brophy CJ, Greenstone MA. How well do we care for patients with end stage chronic obstructive pulmonary disease COPD? *A comparison of palliative care and quality of life in COPD and lung cancer*. Thorax 2000;55(12):1000–6.

7. Murray S, Kendall M, Boyd K *et al*. Illness trajectories and palliative care. *British Medical Journal* 2005;330(7498):1007–11.

8. Lunney J, Lynn J, Foley D *et al*. Patterns of functional decline at the end-of-life. *The Journal of the American Medical Association* 2003;289(18):2387–92.

9. Kamphuisen PW, Agnelli G, Sebastianelli M. Prevention of venous thromboembolism after acute ischemic stroke. *Journal of Thrombosis and Haemostasis* 2005;3(6):1187–94.

10. Geerts W, Pineo G, Heit J *et al*. Prevention of venous thromboembolism: the Seventh ACCP Conference on Antithrombotic and Thrombolytic Therapy. *Chest* 2004;126(3 Suppl):338S–400S.

11. Oger E, Bressollette L, Nonent M *et al*. High prevalence of asymptomatic deep vein thrombosis on admission in a medical unit among elderly patients. *Thrombosis and Haemostasis* 2002;88(4):592–7.

12. Leizorovicz A, Cohen A, Turpie AG *et al*. Randomized, placebo-controlled trial of dalteparin for the prevention of venous thromboembolism in acutely ill medical patients. *Circulation* 2004;110(7):874–9.

13. Cohen A, Davidson B, Gallus A et al. Efficacy and safety of fondaparinux for the prevention of venous thromboembolism in older acute medical patients: randomised placebo controlled trial. *British Medical Journal* 2006;332(7537):325–9.

14. Samama MM, Cohen AT, Darmon JY et al. A comparison of enoxaparin with placebo for the prevention of venous thromboembolism in acutely ill medical patients Prophylaxis in Medical Patients with Enoxaparin Study Group. *The New England Journal of Medicine* 1999;341(11):793–800.

15. Risk and prophylaxis for venous thrombosis in hospital patients. Thromboembolic Risk Factors (THRIFT) Consensus Group. British Medical Journal 1992;305:567–74.

16. Freudenberger R, Hellkamp A, Halperin J et al. Risk of thromboembolism in heart failure: an analysis from the Sudden Cardiac Death in Heart Failure Trial SCD-HeFT. *Circulation* 2007;115(20):2637–41.

17. Goldhaber SZ, Savage DD, Garrison RJ et al. Risk factors for pulmonary embolism The Framingham Study. *The American Journal of Medicine* 1983;74(6):1023–8.

18. Roberts WC, Siegel RJ, McManus BM. Idiopathic dilated cardiomyopathy: analysis of 152 necropsy patients. *The American Journal of Cardiology* 1987;60(16):1340–55.

19. Darze E, Latado A, Guimarães A et al. Incidence and clinical predictors of pulmonary embolism in severe heart failure patients admitted to a coronary care unit. *Chest* 2005;128(4):2576–80.

20. Beemath A, Stein P, Skaf E et al. Risk of venous thromboembolism in patients hospitalized with heart failure. *The American Journal of Cardiology* 2006;98(6):793–5.

21. Beemath A, Skaf E, Stein P. Pulmonary embolism as a cause of death in adults who died with heart failure. *The American Journal of Cardiology* 2006;98(8):1073–5.

22. Attems J, Arbes S, Böhm G et al. The clinical diagnostic accuracy rate regarding the immediate cause of death in a hospitalized geriatric population; an autopsy study of 1594 patients. *Wiener Medizinische Wochenschrift* 2004;154(7–8):159–62.

23. Schonhofer B, D K. Prevalence of deep vein thrombosis of the leg in patients with an acute exacerbation of chronic obstructive pulmonary disease. *Respiration* 1998;65:173–7.

24. Akgun M, Meral M, Onbas O et al. Comparison of clinical characteristics and outcomes of patients with COPD exacerbation with or without venous thromboembolism. *Respiration* 2006;73(4):428–33.

25. Fraisse F, Holzapfel L, Couland JM et al. Nadroparin in the prevention of deep vein thrombosis in acute decompensated COPD The Association of Non-University Affiliated Intensive Care Specialist Physicians of France. *American Journal of Respiratory and Critical Care Medicine* 2000;161(4 Pt 1):1109–14.

26. Winter JH, Buckler PW, Bautista AP et al. Frequency of venous thrombosis in patients with an exacerbation of chronic obstructive lung disease. *Thorax* 1983;38(8):605–8.

27. Tillie-Leblond I, Marquette C, Perez T et al. Pulmonary embolism in patients with unexplained exacerbation of chronic obstructive pulmonary disease: prevalence and risk factors. *Annals of Internal Medicine* 2006;144(6):390–6.

28. Rutschmann O, Cornuz J, Poletti P et al. Should pulmonary embolism be suspected in exacerbation of chronic obstructive pulmonary disease? *Thorax* 2007;62(2):121–5.

29. Zielinski J, MacNee W, Wedzicha J *et al*. Causes of death in patients with COPD and chronic respiratory failure. *Monaldi Archives for Chest Disease* 1997;52(1):43–7.

30. André C, de Freitas GR, Fukujima MM. Prevention of deep venous thrombosis and pulmonary embolism following stroke: a systematic review of published articles. *European Journal of Neurology* 2007;14(1):21–32.

31. Kelly J, Rudd A, Lewis RR *et al*. Venous thromboembolism after acute ischemic stroke: a prospective study using magnetic resonance direct thrombus imaging. *Stroke* 2004;35(10):2320–5.

32. Dickmann U, Voth E, Schicha H *et al*. Heparin therapy, deep-vein thrombosis and pulmonary embolism after intracerebral hemorrhage. *Klinische Wochenschrift* 1988;66(23):1182–3.

33. Viitanen M, Winblad B, Asplund K. Autopsy-verified causes of death after stroke. *Acta Medica Scandinavica* 1987;222(5):401–8.

34. Wiesholzer M, Kitzwögerer M, Harm F *et al*. Prevalence of preterminal pulmonary thromboembolism among patients on maintenance hemodialysis treatment before and after introduction of recombinant erythropoietin. *American Journal of Kidney Diseases* 1999;33(4):702–8.

35. Qureshi M, Cudkowicz M, Zhang H *et al*. Increased incidence of deep venous thrombosis in ALS. *Neurology* 2007;68(1):76–7.

36. Elman LB, Siderowf A, Houseman G *et al*. Venous thrombosis in an ALS population over four years. *Amyotrophic Lateral Sclerosis and Other Motor Neuron Disorders* 2005;6(4):246–9.

37. Samama MM. An epidemiologic study of risk factors for deep vein thrombosis in medical outpatients: the Sirius study. *Archives of Internal Medicine* 2000;160(22):3415–20.

38. Alikhan R, Cohen A, Combe S *et al*. Risk factors for venous thromboembolism in hospitalized patients with acute medical illness: analysis of the MEDENOX Study. *Archives of Internal Medicine* 2004;164(9):963–8.

39. Rosendaal FR. Venous thrombosis: a multicausal disease. *Lancet* 1999;353(9159):1167–73.

40. Anderson F, Spencer F. Risk factors for venous thromboembolism. *Circulation* 2003;107(Suppl 1):I9–16.

41. Howell MD, Geraci JM, Knowlton AA. Congestive heart failure and outpatient risk of venous thromboembolism: a retrospective, case-control study. *Journal of Clinical Epidemiology* 2001;54(8):810–6.

42. Ambrosetti M, Ageno W, Spanevello A *et al*. Prevalence and prevention of venous thromboembolism in patients with acute exacerbations of COPD. *Thrombosis Research* 2003;112(4):203–7.

43. Hansson PO, Eriksson H, Welin L *et al*. Smoking and abdominal obesity: risk factors for venous thromboembolism among middle-aged men: the study of men born in 1913. *Archives of Internal Medicine* 1999;159(16):1886–90.

44. Goldhaber SZ, Grodstein F, Stampfer MJ *et al*. A prospective study of risk factors for pulmonary embolism in women. *The Journal of the American Medical Association* 1997;277(8):642–5.

45. Glynn R, Rosner B. Comparison of risk factors for the competing risks of coronary heart disease, stroke, and venous thromboembolism. *The American Journal of Epidemiology* 2005;162(10):975–82.

46. Hillbom M, Erilä T, Sotaniemi K *et al*. Enoxaparin vs heparin for prevention of deep-vein thrombosis in acute ischaemic stroke: a randomized, double-blind study. *Acta Neurologica Scandinavica* 2002;106(2):84–92.

47. Kelly J, Hunt BJ, Lewis RR *et al*. Dehydration and venous thromboembolism after acute stroke. *The Quarterly Journal of Medicine* 2004;97(5):293–6.

48. Gregory P, Kuhlemeier K. Prevalence of venous thromboembolism in acute hemorrhagic and thromboembolic stroke. *American Journal of Physical Medicine and Rehabilitation* 2003;82(5):364–9.

49. Roth EJ, Lovell L, Harvey RL *et al*. Incidence of and risk factors for medical complications during stroke rehabilitation. *Stroke* 2001;32(2):523–9.

50. Monreal M, Falgá C, Valle R *et al*. Venous thromboembolism in patients with renal insufficiency: findings from the RIETE Registry. *The American Journal of Medicine* 2006;119(12):1073–9.

51. Tveit D, Hypolite I, Hshieh P *et al*. Chronic dialysis patients have high risk for pulmonary embolism. *The American Journal of Kidney Diseases* 2002;39(5):1011–7.

52. Casserly LF, Reddy SM, Dember LM. Venous thromboembolism in end-stage renal disease. *The American Journal of Kidney Diseases* 2000;36(2):405–11.

53. Stolz E, Klötzsch C, Schlachetzki F *et al*. High-dose corticosteroid treatment is associated with an increased risk of developing cerebral venous thrombosis. *European Neurology* 2003;49(4):247–8.

54. Frank R, Altenwerth B, Brandenburg V *et al*. Effect of intravenous high-dose methylprednisolone on coagulation and fibrinolysis markers. *Thrombosis and Haemostasis* 2005;94(2):467–8.

55. Closse C, Seigneur M, Renard M *et al*. Influence of hypoxia and hypoxia-reoxygenation on endothelial P- selectin expression. *Thrombosis Research* 1997;85(2):159–64.

56. Falati S, Liu Q, Gross P *et al*. Accumulation of tissue factor into developing thrombi in vivo is dependent upon microparticle P-selectin glycoprotein ligand 1 and platelet P-selectin. *The Journal of Experimental Medicine* 2003;197(11):1585–98.

57. Paulus WJ. Cytokines and heart failure. *Heart Failure Monitor* 2000;1(2):50–6.

58. Biemond BJ, Levi M, Ten C *et al*. Plasminogen activator and plasminogen activator inhibitor I release during experimental endotoxaemia in chimpanzees: effect of interventions in the cytokine and coagulation cascades. *Clinical Science* 1995;88(5):587–94.

59. Parry GC, Mackman N. Transcriptional regulation of tissue factor expression in human endothelial cells. Arteriosclerosis, *Thrombosis, and Vascular Biology* 1995;15(5):612–21.

60. Chong A, Lip GH. Viewpoint: the prothrombotic state in heart failure: a maladaptive inflammatory response? *European Journal of Heart Failure* 2007;9(2):124–8.

61. Sbarouni E, Bradshaw A, Andreotti F *et al*. Relationship between hemostatic abnormalities and neuroendocrine activity in heart failure. *American Heart Journal* 1994;127(3):607–12.

62. Moyses C, Cederholm WA, Michel CC. Haemoconcentration and accumulation of white cells in the feet during venous stasis. *International Journal of Microcirculation, Clinical and Experimental* 1987;5(4):311–20.

63. Tapson V. The role of smoking in coagulation and thromboembolism in chronic obstructive pulmonary disease. *Proceedings of the American Thoracic Society* 2005;2(1):71–7.

64. Mendall MA, Patel P, Asante M *et al*. Relation of serum cytokine concentrations to cardiovascular risk factors and coronary heart disease. *Heart* 1997;78(3):273–7.

65. Cermak J, Key NS, Bach RR *et al*. C-reactive protein induces human peripheral blood monocytes to synthesize tissue factor. *Blood* 1993;82(2):513–20.

66. Newby DE, Wright RA, Dawson P *et al*. The L-arginine/nitric oxide pathway contributes to the acute release of tissue plasminogen activator in vivo in man. *Cardiovascular Research* 1998;38(2):485–92.

67. Erelel M, Cuhadaroglu C, Ece T *et al*. The frequency of deep venous thrombosis and pulmonary embolus in acute exacerbation of chronic obstructive pulmonary disease. *Respiratory Medicine* 2002;96(7):515–18.

68. Vayá A, Mira Y, Martìnez M *et al*. Biological risk factors for deep vein thrombosis. *Clinical Hemorheology and Microcirculation* 2002;26(1):41–53.

69. Cadroy Y, Hanson SR. Effects of red blood cell concentration on hemostasis and thrombus formation in a primate model. *Blood* 1990;75(11):2185–93.

70. Casserly L, Dember L. Thrombosis in end-stage renal disease. *Seminars in Dialysis* 2003;16(3):245–56.

71. Kakkar VV, Howe CT, Flanc C *et al*. Natural history of postoperative deep-vein thrombosis. *Lancet* 1969;2(7614):230–2.

72. Fitzmaurice D, Murray E. Thromboprophylaxis for adults in hospital. *British Medical Journal* 2007;334(7602):1017–18.

73. Kearon C. Natural history of venous thromboembolism. *Circulation* 2003;107(Suppl 1):I22–30.

74. Stein PD, Henry JW, Relyea B. Untreated patients with pulmonary embolism Outcome, clinical, and laboratory assessment. *Chest* 1995;107(4):931–5.

75. Monreal M, Kakkar AK, Caprini JA *et al*. The outcome after treatment of venous thromboembolism is different in surgical and acutely ill medical patients Findings from the RIETE registry. *Journal of Thrombosis and Haemostasis* 2004;2(11):1892–8.

76. Monreal M, Muñoz T, Naraine V *et al*. Pulmonary embolism in patients with chronic obstructive pulmonary disease or congestive heart failure. *The American Journal of Medicine* 2006;119(10):851–8.

77. Carson JL, Terrin ML, Duff A *et al*. Pulmonary embolism and mortality in patients with COPD. *Chest* 1996;110(5):1212–19.

78. Holmström M, Lindmarker P, Granqvist S *et al*. A 6-month venographic follow-up in 164 patients with acute deep vein thrombosis. *Thrombosis and Haemostasis* 1997;78(2):803–7.

79. Prandoni P, Lensing AW, Cogo A *et al*. The long-term clinical course of acute deep venous thrombosis. *Annals of Internal Medicine* 1996;125(1):1–7.

80. Brandjes DP, Büller HR, Heijboer H *et al*. Randomised trial of effect of compression stockings in patients with symptomatic proximal-vein thrombosis. *Lancet* 1997;349(9054):759–62.

81. Prandoni P, Lensing AW, Prins MR. Long-term outcomes after deep venous thrombosis of the lower extremities. *Vascular Medicine* 1998;3(1):57–60.

82. Prandoni P, Lensing AA, Prins M et al. Below-knee elastic compression stockings to prevent the post- thrombotic syndrome: a randomized, controlled trial. *Annals of Internal Medicine* 2004;141(4):249–56.

83. Ginsberg JS, Magier D, Mackinnon B et al. Intermittent compression units for severe post-phlebitic syndrome: a randomized crossover study. *Canadian Medical Association Journal* 1999;160(9):1303–6.

84. Kahn S, Hirsch A, Shrier I. Effect of postthrombotic syndrome on health-related quality of life after deep venous thrombosis. *Archives of Internal Medicine* 2002;162(10):1144–8.

85. Kahn S. The post-thrombotic syndrome: the forgotten morbidity of deep venous thrombosis. *Journal of Thrombosis and Thrombolysis* 2006;21(1):41–8.

86. Cornwall JV, Doré CJ, Lewis JD. Leg ulcers: epidemiology and aetiology. *British Journal of Surgery* 1986;73(9):693–6.

87. Pengo V, Lensing AA, Prins M et al. Incidence of chronic thromboembolic pulmonary hypertension after pulmonary embolism. *The New England Journal of Medicine* 2004;350(22):2257–64.

88. Cramer S, Rordorf G, Maki J et al. Increased pelvic vein thrombi in cryptogenic stroke: results of the Paradoxical Emboli from Large Veins in Ischemic Stroke PELVIS study. *Stroke* 2004;35(1):46–50.

89. Khairy P, O'Donnell C, Landzberg M. Transcatheter closure versus medical therapy of patent foramen ovale and presumed paradoxical thromboemboli: a systematic review. *Annals of Internal Medicine* 2003;139(9):753–60.

90. Stein P, Beemath A, Meyers F et al. Pulmonary embolism and deep venous thrombosis in hospitalized adults with chronic obstructive pulmonary disease. *Journal of Cardiovascular Medicine* (Hagerstown, MD) 2007;8(4):253–7.

91. Lesser BA, Leeper KVJ, Stein PD et al. The diagnosis of acute pulmonary embolism in patients with chronic obstructive pulmonary disease. *Chest* 1992;102(1):17–22.

92. Wagner PD, Dantzker DR, Dueck R et al. Ventilation-perfusion inequality in chronic obstructive pulmonary disease. *The Journal of Clinical Investigation* 1977;59(2):203–16.

93. Meignan M, Simonneau G, Oliveira L et al. Computation of ventilation-perfusion ratio with Kr-81m in pulmonary embolism. *Journal of Nuclear Medicine* 1984;25(2):149–55.

94. Hartmann IJ, Hagen PJ, Melissant CF et al. Diagnosing acute pulmonary embolism: effect of chronic obstructive pulmonary disease on the performance of D-dimer testing, ventilation /perfusion scintigraphy, spiral computed tomographic angiography, and conventional angiography ANTELOPE Study Group Advances in New Technologies Evaluating the Localization of Pulmonary Embolism. *American Journal of Respiratory and Critical Care Medicine* 2000;162(6):2232–7.

95. Sohne M, Kruip MJHA, Nijkeuter M et al. Accuracy of clinical decision rule, D-dimer and spiral computed tomography in patients with malignancy, previous venous thromboembolism, COPD or heart failure and in older patients with suspected pulmonary embolism. *Journal of Thrombosis and Haemostasis* 2006;4(5):1042–6.

96. Chaudhuri GX, Costa JL. Clinical findings associated with pulmonary embolism in a rehabilitation setting. *Archives of Physical Medicine and Rehabilitation* 1991;72(9):671–3.

97. Kelly J, Hunt B, Rudd A *et al.* Pulmonary embolism and pneumonia may be confounded after acute stroke and may co-exist. *Age and Ageing* 2002;31(4):235–9.

98. Goldhaber SZ, Hennekens CH, Evans DA *et al.* Factors associated with correct antemortem diagnosis of major pulmonary embolism. *The American Journal of Medicine* 1982;73(6):822–6.

99. Murray HW, Ellis GC, Blumenthal DS *et al.* Fever and pulmonary thromboembolism. *The American Journal of Medicine* 1979;67(2):232–5.

100. Wells PS, Holbrook AM, Crowther NR *et al.* Interactions of warfarin with drugs and food. *Annals of Internal Medicine* 1994;121(9):676–83.

101. Landefeld CS, Beyth RJ. Anticoagulant-related bleeding: clinical epidemiology, prediction, and prevention. *The American Journal of Medicine* 1993;95(3):315–28.

102. Beyth RJ, Quinn LM, Landefeld CS. Prospective evaluation of an index for predicting the risk of major bleeding in outpatients treated with warfarin. *The American Journal of Medicine* 1998;105(2):91–9.

103. Nieuwenhuis HK, Albada J, Banga JD *et al.* Identification of risk factors for bleeding during treatment of acute venous thromboembolism with heparin or low molecular weight heparin. *Blood* 1991;78(9):2337–43.

104. Dentali F, Douketis J, Lim W *et al.* Combined aspirin-oral anticoagulant therapy compared with oral anticoagulant therapy alone among patients at risk for cardiovascular disease: a meta-analysis of randomized trials. *Archives of Internal Medicine* 2007;167(2):117–24.

105. Baker RN, Broward JA, Fang HC *et al.* Anticoagulant therapy of cerebral infarction: report of a national cooperative study. *Research Publications – Association for Research in Nervous and Mental Disease* 1966;41:287–302.

106. Enger E, Boyesen S. Long-term anticoagulant therapy in patients with cerebral infarction A crontrolled clinical study. *Acta Medica Scandinavica. Supplementum* 1965;438:1–61.

107. Gubitz G, Sandercock P, Counsell C. Anticoagulants for acute ischaemic stroke. *Cochrane Database of Systematic Reviews* 2004;3:CD000024.

108. Bath PM, Lindenstrom E, Boysen G *et al.* Tinzaparin in acute ischaemic stroke TAIST: a randomised aspirin- controlled trial. *Lancet* 2001;358(9283):702–10.

109. Landefeld CS, Cook EF, Flatley M *et al.* Identification and preliminary validation of predictors of major bleeding in hospitalized patients starting anticoagulant therapy. *The American Journal of Medicine* 1987;82(4):703–13.

110. Petitti DB, Strom BL, Melmon KL. Prothrombin time ratio and other factors associated with bleeding in patients treated with warfarin. *Journal of Clinical Epidemiology* 1989;42(8):759–64.

111. Vieweg WV, Piscatelli RL, Houser JJ *et al.* Complications of intravenous administration of heparin in elderly women. *The Journal of the American Medical Association* 1970;213(8):1303–6.

112. Walker AM, Jick H. Predictors of bleeding during heparin therapy. *The Journal of the American Medical Association* 1980;244(11):1209–12.

113. Eikelboom J, Ginsberg J, Hirsh J. Anticoagulation for venous thromboembolism. *British Medical Journal* 2007;334(7595):645.

114. Lee AY, Hirsh J. Diagnosis and treatment of venous thromboembolism. *Annual Review of Medicine* 2002;53:15–33.

115. Campbell IA, Bentley DP, Prescott RJ *et al.* Anticoagulation for three versus six months in patients with deep vein thrombosis or pulmonary embolism, or both: randomised trial. *British Medical Journal* 2007;334(7595):674.

116. Goldhaber S, Turpie AG. Prevention of venous thromboembolism among hospitalized medical patients. *Circulation* 2005;111(1):e1.

117. Leizorovicz A, Mismetti P. Preventing venous thromboembolism in medical patients. *Circulation* 2004;110(Suppl 1):IV13–9.

118. Hill J, Treasure T. Reducing the risk of venous thromboembolism deep vein thrombosis and pulmonary embolism in inpatients having surgery: summary of NICE guidance. *British Medical Journal* 2007;334(7602):1053–4.

119. Dentali F, Douketis J, Gianni M *et al.* Meta-analysis: anticoagulant prophylaxis to prevent symptomatic venous thromboembolism in hospitalized medical patients. *Annals of Internal Medicine* 2007;146(4):278–88.

120. Belch JJ, Lowe GD, Ward AG *et al.* Prevention of deep vein thrombosis in medical patients by low-dose heparin. *Scottish Medical Journal* 1981;26(2):115–17.

121. Dahan R, Houlbert D, Caulin C *et al.* Prevention of deep vein thrombosis in elderly medical in-patients by a low molecular weight heparin: a randomized double-blind trial. *Haemostasis* 1986;16(2):159–64.

122. Gärdlund B. Randomised controlled trial of low-dose heparin for prevention of fatal pulmonary embolism in patients with infectious diseases. The Heparin Prophylaxis Study Group. *Lancet* 1996;347:1357–61.

123. Mahé I, Bergmann JF, d'Azémar P *et al.* Lack of effect of a low-molecular-weight heparin nadroparin on mortality in bedridden medical in-patients: a prospective randomised double-blind study. *European Journal of Clinical Pharmacology* 2005;61(5–6):347–51.

124. Lederle F, Sacks J, Fiore L *et al.* The prophylaxis of medical patients for thromboembolism pilot study. *The American Journal of Medicine* 2006;119(1):54–9.

125. Sherman D, Albers G, Bladin C *et al.* The efficacy and safety of enoxaparin versus unfractionated heparin for the prevention of venous thromboembolism after acute ischaemic stroke PREVAIL Study: an open-label randomised comparison. *Lancet* 2007;369(9570):1347–55.

126. Mismetti P, Laporte S, Tardy B *et al.* Prevention of venous thromboembolism in internal medicine with unfractionated or low-molecular-weight heparins: a meta-analysis of randomised clinical trials. *Thrombosis and Haemostasis* 2000;83(1):14–9.

127. Kleber FX, Witt C, Vogel G *et al.* Randomized comparison of enoxaparin with unfractionated heparin for the prevention of venous thromboembolism in medical patients with heart failure or severe respiratory disease. *American Heart Journal* 2003;145(4):614–21.

128. Sandercock P, Counsell C, Stobbs SL. Low-molecular-weight heparins or heparinoids versus standard unfractionated heparin for acute ischaemic stroke. *Cochrane Database of Systematic Reviews* 2005(2):CD000119.

129. Kamphuisen P, Agnelli G. What is the optimal pharmacological prophylaxis for the prevention of deep-vein thrombosis and pulmonary embolism in patients with acute ischemic stroke? *Thrombosis Research* 2007;119(3):265–74.

130. Burleigh E, Wang C, Foster D *et al*. Thromboprophylaxis in medically ill patients at risk for venous thromboembolism. *American Journal of Health-System Pharmacy* 2006;63(Suppl 6):S23–9.

131. Sandercock P, Dennis M. Venous thromboembolism after acute stroke. *Stroke* 2001;32(6):1443–8.

132. Collaborative overview of randomised controlled trials of antiplatelet therapy III: reduction in venous thrombosis and pulmonary embolism by antiplatelet prophylaxis among surgical and medical patients. Antiplatelet Trialists' Collaboration. *British Medical Journal* 1994;308:235–46.

133. Gubitz G, Sandercock P, Counsell C. Antiplatelet therapy for acute ischaemic stroke. *Cochrane Database of Systematic Reviews* 2000(2):CD000029.

134. Prevention of pulmonary embolism and deep vein thrombosis with low-dose aspirin. PEP Trial Collaborative Group. *Lancet* 2000;355:1295–302.

135. McKenna R, Galante J, Bachmann F *et al*. Prevention of venous thromboembolism after total knee replacement by high-dose aspirin or intermittent calf and thigh compression. *British Medical Journal* 1980;280(6213):514–17.

136. Westrich GH, Sculco TP. Prophylaxis against deep venous thrombosis after total knee arthroplasty Pneumatic plantar compression and aspirin compared with aspirin alone. The Journal of Bone and Joint Surgery. *American Volume* 1996;78(6):826–34.

137. Albers G, Amarenco P, Easton J *et al*. Antithrombotic and thrombolytic therapy for ischemic stroke: the Seventh ACCP Conference on Antithrombotic and Thrombolytic Therapy. *Chest* 2004;126(3 Suppl):483S–512S.

138. Amaragiri SV, Lees TA. Elastic compression stockings for prevention of deep vein thrombosis. *Cochrane Database of Systematic Reviews* 2000(3):CD001484.

139. Muir KW, Watt A, Baxter G *et al*. Randomized trial of graded compression stockings for prevention of deep-vein thrombosis after acute stroke. *The Quarterly Journal of Medicine* 2000;93(6):359–64.

140. Noble SIR, Nelson A, Turner C *et al*. Acceptability of low molecular weight heparin thromboprophylaxis for inpatients receiving palliative care: qualitative study. *British Medical Journal* 2006;332(7541):577–80.

141. Lippi G, Guidi G. Thromboprophylaxis in stroke patients. *Stroke* 2005;36(10):2067–8.

142. Mazzone C, Chiodo G, Sandercock P *et al*. Physical methods for preventing deep vein thrombosis in stroke. *Cochrane Database of Systematic Reviews* 2004(4):CD001922.

143. Rashid ST, Thursz MR, Razvi NA *et al*. Venous thromboprophylaxis in UK medical inpatients. *Journal of the Royal Society of Medicine* 2005;98(11):507–12.

144. Elis A, Ellis MH. Preventing venous thromboembolism in acute medical patients. *The Quarterly Journal of Medicine* 2004;97(12):797–801.

145. Stark J, Kilzer W. Venous thromboembolic prophylaxis in hospitalized medical patients. *The Annals of Pharmacotherapy* 2004;38(1):36–40.

146. Cohen AT. Venous thromboembolic disease management of the nonsurgical moderate- and high-risk patient. *Seminars in Hematology* 2000;37(Suppl 5):19–22.

147. Eldor A. Applying risk assessment models in non-surgical patients: effective risk stratification. *Blood Coagulation and Fibrinolysis* 1999;10(Suppl 2):S91–7.

148. Davidson BL. Applying risk assessment models in non-surgical patients: overview of our clinical experience. *Blood Coagulation and Fibrinolysis* 1999;10(Suppl 2):S85–9.

149. Yale SH, Medlin SC, Liang H *et al*. Risk assessment model for venothromboembolism in post-hospitalized patients. *International Angiology* 2005;24(3):250–4.

150. Cohen A, Alikhan R, Arcelus J *et al*. Assessment of venous thromboembolism risk and the benefits of thromboprophylaxis in medical patients. *Thrombosis and Haemostasis* 2005;94(4):750–9.

151. Caprini JA, Arcelus JI, Reyna JJ. Effective risk stratification of surgical and nonsurgical patients for venous thromboembolic disease. *Seminars in Hematology* 2001;38(Suppl 5):12–9.

152. Jubb AM. Palliative care research: trading ethics for an evidence base. *Journal of Medical Ethics* 2002;28(6):342–6.

153. Grande GE, Todd CJ. Why are trials in palliative care so difficult? *Palliative Medicine* 2000;14(1):69–74.

154. Noble SR, Finlay IG. Is long-term low-molecular-weight heparin acceptable to palliative care patients in the treatment of cancer related venous thromboembolism? A qualitative study. *Palliative Medicine* 2005;19(3):197–201.

155. Chambers J. Prophylactic heparin in palliative care: to a challenging idea. *British Medical Journal* 2006;332(7543):729.

156. Kelly J, Rudd T, Lewis R *et al*. Mortality from pulmonary embolism after acute stroke: can we do better? *Age and Ageing* 2002;31(3):159-61.

157. Kelly J, Rudd A, Lewis R, *et al*. The relationship between acute ischaemic stroke and plasma D-dimer levels in patients developing neither venous thromboembolism nor major intercurrent illness. *Blood Coagulation and Fibrinolysis* 2003;14(7):639-45.

158. Kelly J, Rudd A, Lewis RR *et al*. Screening for proximal deep vein thrombosis after acute ischemic stroke: a prospective study using clinical factors and plasma D-dimers. *Journal of Thrombosis and Haemostasis* 2004;2(8):1321–6.

159. Wilson R, Murray P. Cost-effectiveness of screening for deep vein thrombosis by ultrasound at admission to stroke rehabilitation. *Archives of Physical Medicine and Rehabilitation* 2005;86(10):1941–8.

Index